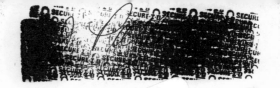

Your Body Believes
Every Word You Say

by
Barbara Hoberman Levine

Published by

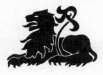

Aslan Publishing
310 Blue Ridge Drive
Boulder Creek, CA 95006

For a free catalog of other books by Aslan Publishing,
please send a stamped, self-addressed envelope to:

Aslan Publishing
310 Blue Ridge Drive
Boulder Creek, CA 95006
(408) 338-7504

IMPORTANT NOTE TO READERS:
The suggestions in this book for personal healing and growth are not meant to
substitute for the advice of a trained professional such as a medical doctor or
psychiatrist. It is essential to consult such a professional in the case of any physical or mental symptoms. The publishers and author expressly disclaim any lia-
bility for injuries resulting from use by readers of the methods contained herein.

Levine, Barbara Hoberman, 1937-
    Your body believes every word you say.

    Includes bibliographical references.
    1. Health. 2. Mind and body. 3. Emotions--Health
aspects. 4. Sick--language. I. Title
RA776.L646 1991   616'.0019   90-1169
ISBN 0-944031-07-2

Excerpts reprinted from *Healing From Within* by Dennis T. Jaffe. Copyright © 1980 by
Dennis T. Jaffe. Reprinted by permission of Alfred A. Knopf, Inc.
Excerpts reprinted from *Minding the Body, Mending the Mind* by Joan Borysenko, ©
1987 by Joan Borysenko. Reprinted with permission of Addison-Wesley Publishing Co.,
Inc. Reading, Massachusetts.
Excerpts reprinted from *Brain/Mind Bulletin* published by Marilyn Ferguson, Box 42211,
Los Angeles, CA 90042, USA.
Excerpts reprinted from *Superimmunity* by Paul Pearsall, Ph.D. Copyright © 1987 by Paul
Pearsall. Reprinted with permission of McGraw-Hill Publishing Co., New York

Book design by Dawson Church
Cover design by Brenda Plowman
Printed in USA
First Edition
10 9 8 7 6 5 4 3 2 1

This book is joyously dedicated to my family
for loving me unconditionally, through thick and thin,
no matter what I said or did.

To my wonderful husband, Harold Levine;
To my terrific sister, Arlene Hoberman Kyler;
To my dear children,
Jennifer, Steven, and Kenneth Levine;
To Kenneth's great wife, Linda Rozans, and their child,
my precious granddaughter, Rachel Anne Levine.

Foreword

Barbara does an enlightening and entertaining job of illustrating how the words and images we use in our daily expression of life can be metaphors for our health status. More importantly, she shows how we can change the course of illness and dysfunction by becoming more aware of, and choosing more carefully, those words and images. Perhaps the most significant "discovery" of the late twentieth century is the realization that our attitudes and beliefs shape our perceptions and our lives, and that we can become aware of and change these perceptions, producing profound effects on the physical body.

She also points out that utilization of relaxation and visualization techniques can greatly improve the effectiveness of conventional medical treatment. This has been verified in my clinical experience. Many proponents of innovative techniques cast medicine as a potential adversary. Barbara shows how empowered patients can be speeded to healing by working closely with the medical establishment while developing a keen sensitivity to their own inner process. This book shows that patients who "take charge" of their images and attitudes, and don't fall into the trap of helplessness and victimhood, can speed their recovery during treatment. Also, evoking the "story" of their illness or dysfunction usually reframes their experiences and moves them to a place of greater inner power.

Cheers to Barbara for a helpful and empowering book!

Emmett E. Miller, M.D.

Acknowledgments

So many people supported me in writing this book since I began in 1983. You have my thanks even if I don't mention your name. I love you all and wish you the best.

Special thanks to W.C. Ellerbroek, M.D., recently deceased, whose ideas sparked my own and who so generously shared his thoughts with me. Special thanks and big hugs to Bernie Siegel, M.D., and Emmett Miller, M.D., both of whom went out of their way to encourage me from the earliest stages of my work on this book. Their belief in me helped me to believe in myself and encouraged me to ask for help from the rest of the health community.

Thanks for editorial contributions from therapists Linda Zelizer, Eric Esselstyn, Roberta Tager, Dorothy Thau, Julia Bondi, Alice Katz, Jack Henry, Denny Cooper, Ananda Saha, Debbie Blair, Ted Smith; M.D.s Vincent Scavo, Bob Lang, Harry Brown, and Montague Ullman; chiropractors Robert Marshall and Jackie Ruzga; naturopaths Larry Caprio and Marvin Schweitzer; optometrist Carl Gruning; physicist Buryl Payne; dentist Mark Breiner. In addition to those doctors already mentioned, thanks to Drs. Abrams, Burd, Bushell, Cohen, Dogali, Epstein, Gill, Hankin, Hu, Kauders, Kunkes, Levin, Levy, Lipow, Reichgut, Sachs, and Sasaki for unswerving support during the years of my research.

Thanks to graduate school teachers Ruth Gonchar Brennan, Jackie Rinaldi, Barry Tarshis, Ted Cheney, Jim Keenan, and Joe Cahalan, who, among others, nurtured my writing and communications skills; to writer friends Liz Goldner, Melissa Schnirring, Michael Mesmer, Howie Sann, Judy Berkun, and Nadine Fauerbach, who read early versions of the manuscript and offered suggestions for improvement; to Judy Glaser for the "human as instrument" analogy; to Susan Flaster and to Myrin Borysenko, whose good words came just when I needed them most; to Marilyn Ferguson for being a role model and sharing the information in *Brain/Mind Bulletin*. To agent Adele Leone for introducing me to Aslan Publishing—Brenda Plowman and Dawson Church are the best publishers a first-time author can have. To Jenny D'Angelo for sending love the whole time she was copyediting the book. To Michael Karpilow for proving that I am photogenic. To The Great Tradition sales representatives for "remembering me."

Major credit goes to my editors. Marcia Yudkin guided and encouraged me through every revision. Her belief in me and her sensitivity to the material was absolutely crucial. Dawson Church took over and pushed and prodded me, ever so gently, until finally we both knew we had the book we wanted.

For inspiration and information thanks to Werner Erhard, Stewart Emery, John-Roger, John Graham, Henry Reed, and John Bear. To Gene and Eva Graf, Baba Muktananda, Gurumayi Chidvilasananda, Acharya Sushil Kumar Muni Ji, Rabbi Arnold Sher, Grace 'n Vessels of Christ, Kenneth Copeland, and my many prayer partners—for spiritual sustenance, information, and growth.

With gratitude to all my former students and teachers from whom I learned so much. To the rest of my friends and family for always backing me with unconditional loving care. To Jean Swilling, Irma Lesser, Debby Masone, Gemma Abboud, Terry Caprio, John and Jane Mather, Ruth and Jack Levine, Jo Willard, Lois O'Brien, Tony Storace, Ray Tata, Mary and John Steinmetz, John Moretti, Judi Rosner, Lele Stephens, Gail Cohen, Ruth Casl, Lydia Dixon, Elly Davidson, and Jim Bacik for being there when I needed them. To The Women's Bliss Group for seen and unseen support. And to the unknown readers who will benefit from this work.

To my parents, Abraham and Evelyn Estrin Hoberman, now deceased, for giving birth to me and my sister and nurturing us through the early years. Lastly, and most importantly, to the loving God who always watches over me, protects me, and lets me know what to do.

Many blessings,
Barbara Hoberman Levine—June 1990

CONTENTS

SELF-HELP EXPERIENCES

The Brain Tumor: My Growth

Introduction

The ideas in this book arose from the most profound adventure of my life. That life-changing experience seemed to begin in 1970 with the birth of my third child, Jennifer. But looking back, I see the experience actually began in 1966 after both my parents died in their early fifties. This was the biggest shock of my life. I became fearful and depressed, but I wasn't adept at handling or understanding my feelings at that time. Then, after Jennifer's birth, I thought I was perfectly happy. But the stress of the previous four years had affected me.

I developed a weakness in my voice and could barely talk above a whisper. Doctors told me my left vocal cord was paralyzed, but they didn't know why. I was 32 years old. The pain I suffered searching for a diagnosis was almost unbearable, making me feel even sicker. Every test came back negative. A virus was blamed when no one could find another cause. After that I lived in terror—afraid of getting sicker, afraid of taking more tests, not even sure I would live. A year later I became deaf in my left ear. Doctors again blamed a virus.

At that time, I was fat, a heavy smoker, and in poor physical condition. Having a paralyzed left vocal cord and a deaf *left* ear actually helped push me in the *right* direction. I realized I needed to find a way to live longer and healthier, so I could be with my two sons and my new daughter as they grew into adulthood. Seeing my children grow up was always a benchmark event in my mind.

I began to live one day at a time, relieving my fear whenever possible by enjoying some of the good things in my life—a nice family, good friends, and a comfortable home. After a year, my voice began to improve somewhat, even though the paralysis and deafness remained. My fear became more bearable when I focused on my newly found life purpose, which was to perfect my ability to think for myself and help others to do the same. Working for women's rights and learning how to heal myself were key elements in this quest.

When my real growth began, I learned to live each day more fully because I didn't know how much time I had left. By living through each day I might live long enough to see my children grow up. "One day at a time" became a guiding principle in my life.

The need to have a reason is so strong that we blamed my debilitating physical symptoms on viruses for four years. In 1974, after getting myself in shape mentally and physically, I felt I was ready to handle anything that came up. I remember thinking, "Even if I need brain surgery I could handle it now." After more tests I finally received an accurate diagnosis. A biopsy done through my left ear proved I had a rare, slow-growing, non-malignant tumor. I had a *growth in my head*.

No tumor had been found in 1970 (this was before CAT scans) but my growth began then—physically, mentally, emotionally, and spiritually. Notice the multiple meanings of the word "growth." In 1974 a neurosurgeon told me he considered the tumor inoperable, as the potential for brain damage from surgery was too great. The tumor was wrapped around several nerves at the point where they exited my brain, next to the brain stem. It was putting pressure on the cranial nerves, affecting my speech and hearing. But the tumor was benign, slow-growing, and small enough for me to live with. It was a partial relief to finally know the truth.

After this diagnosis, a big question was how to heal myself or at least prevent the tumor from growing. The medical community didn't offer much help beyond one doctor's recommendation to "maybe try radiation treatment." He didn't sound at all convinced that that therapy would help. So I declined, believing that radiation would harm me more than help me. Given what I have learned since then, I know I made the correct decision. *If we believe that a treatment will harm us, it probably will.*

Instead I began using holistic healing techniques: diet, exercise, prayer, meditation, rolfing, massage, and chiropractic. I explored Reiki, polarity, and other energy healing modalities. You name it, I probably tried it. For a year I fasted one day a week on fresh juices, detoxifying my body and improving my health enormously.

When years passed with no new symptoms—I ignored little signs—I told myself I was healed. I thought, "The tumor probably dissolved when I fasted." I didn't have a CAT scan after they became available, perhaps preferring ignorant bliss over the news of an inoperable growth. When a doctor suggested I take X rays to check the status of the tumor, I practically turned and ran. What good would it do me to know? To get through each day, I needed to believe it was gone. I believed in my positive inner growth. I was healthy!

In addition to self-healing, my life revolved around my family and helping others in a variety of ways. I began teaching courses for women about women. Later, as my studies and personal growth continued, I taught communication, meditation, metaphysics, and holistic health courses to both men and women.

In 1971, as president of the local National Organization for Women chapter, I ran a women's sexuality conference. After studying for a non-academic Metaphysical Science degree (M.Sc.), I did private counseling. The form of my work has often changed, but the underlying thread remains the same: I am a communicator, catalyst, consciousness raiser, and networker of people and ideas.

Few people even knew I had a tumor. When my first symptoms appeared in 1970, I felt as though I had been reborn. I was spiritually a new person, thinking differently, seeing through different eyes. I used to joke, "Taking all those diagnostic tests brainwashed me, washing out a lot of bad stuff from my brain." But somehow it was really true and not a joke. I had a new, better life filled with purpose, meaning, and commitment. I was growing spiritually—in faith—and humanly—in my ability to love and serve others.

The idea for this book originated in 1976 while I was working towards my Master of Arts in Communication degree. By that time I felt pretty good, my weight was at a normal level, I exercised daily, and I no longer smoked. I spoke clearly in a new voice, but my hearing loss remained.

I enrolled in a class called "Language and Communication." The purpose of the course was "to clarify the role of speech, language, and thought in making humans human." As I looked for a topic for a term paper, a headline on the cover of *Co-Evolution Quarterly* caught my eye: "Language, Thought and Disease" by W.C. Ellerbroek, M.D. On the cover was this quote: "Acne may result from inaccurate self-reporting and be cured by good semantics." Dr. Ellerbroek confirmed what I was already discovering in my own experience.

All these years I've been my own guinea pig, searching for ways to help myself. I pass on what I learn to others in my role as teacher, counselor, or healer. Writing and talking are two ways to share information. As I talked about these ideas and gave copies of my term paper to people, the ideas expanded. The term "seedthoughts" occurred to me as a convenient summary of the correspondence of language to symptoms. "Seedthoughts" is shorthand for the idea that thoughts affect us physically and emotionally. They can lead to the physical symptoms of disease. Our thoughts are like seeds that we plant in our minds and hearts. When they germinate they produce wellness or illness.

One day, while taking a walk, I realized that I could present my ideas about language and healing in the form of a book. I'd always wanted to write but never knew what to write about; finally this theme seemed perfect. As soon as I imagined a title in my mind, I recognized my mission and purpose in life. Writing became part of my healing process.

I wrote the first draft in 1983–84. At that time I assumed that the tumor was gone or at least removed as a threat to my well-being. For 14 years there had been no major new symptoms. My voice had become stronger, though talking a lot sometimes tired me. I was still deaf on the left but it wasn't all bad: I could hear everything I wanted to hear through my right ear, and a beneficial side effect was literally being able to turn a deaf ear to unwanted communication. Sleeping on my right side led to total quiet.

Writing this book enabled me to know myself better. I recognized that my body expressed my unconscious emotions. For example, I remembered the fears that I began to experience when I first lost my voice and hearing. I wondered which came first, the thought "I lost my nerve" or the loss of the physical nerve energy that resulted from constriction by the tumor. At first I believed that my physical disabilities led to my fearful outlook. My physical condition was—literally and symbolically—an *unnerving* experience.

Today, with the benefit of hindsight, I can see that *my physical condition encouraged me to feel the unconscious emotions and fears already within me.* It enabled me to witness myself being afraid, and with this external dramatization, to realize how fearful I had really always been.

By externalizing unconscious emotions in this way, life-threatening illnesses often lead to changes, which in turn allow emotional and spiritual healing to begin. Losing my nerve—feeling fears and developing phobias—showed me what I needed to face in order to heal my spirit. My disabilities led me to the faith I needed to be able to rely on: Faith in my abilities. Faith in my body and my mind. Faith in my understanding of a loving God, where previously I had seen God as a being to be feared. Such faith coupled with right action may be the best protection any of us has.

In August, 1984, I read about two Connecticut neurosurgeons who were using lasers to remove brain tumors. I thought their techniques made surgery possible in the unlikely event that my growth was still there. I decided to have a CAT scan to prove once and for all that the tumor was gone. But I wasn't really as self-confident as I pretended to be. In case the news might be bad, I put off the fearsome CAT scan till November, so that I could finish writing the first draft of my book. Still, I purposefully left space on a page to add the news that the tumor was gone.

In September I had my first new symptom in years, in the form of pressure which affected my balance. I was literally being "pressed" to take the test. I later learned that the tumor had actually grown larger and was pressing on the brain stem. When I stood up after sitting for a long time, I'd feel a pounding in my head and have difficulty standing straight, until my cerebro-spinal fluid readjusted to my standing up.

The November scan proved the tumor was not gone. In fact, it had become life-threatening. I had no real physical pain, but doctors said I had less than three years to live unless the tumor were surgically removed.

In February, 1985, I underwent eight hours of brain surgery. The tumor was completely removed. My basic recovery was rapid, with just four days spent in intensive care. But as well as pressing on the brain stem, the tumor had been affecting the cranial nerves which transmit neural messages to the body's muscles. I was left disabled, as though I had suffered a stroke. I could hardly talk—there was no sound. Though I was able to think clearly and knew the words to use, my voice was so soft I couldn't be heard. I could barely swallow; I saw double because my eyes didn't focus properly; my face drooped on one side; I couldn't walk alone or balance myself; I used a wheelchair for three months, and my entire left side was weakened.

Fortunately my mind, memory, and intellect remained intact. I managed to keep a journal. My right (writing) hand was okay, and I kept one eye closed in order not to see double. All cranial nerves but the one that governed my tongue remained intact.

My doctors, my family, and I expected that I would come out of surgery healthy and able to resume my life as before. Instead I spent three weeks in Bridgeport Hospital and four weeks at a rehabilitation center.

After coming home my progress speeded up. I soon looked great. Function returned quickly to my facial muscles and I learned to eat almost everything, even with the swallowing problems. My eyes improved after three months. I could read and watch television. More importantly, I could work. I began writing again, eventually completely revising this book.

Everything improved, slowly or rapidly, depending on whose perspective is involved. For a time I walked a bit like a wobbling toddler or a staggering drunk. I still carry a cane when I walk in the woods or during snowy, icy weather. Typing is difficult because my left side isn't well-coordinated. In 1987 I had another operation which strengthened my voice by allowing my right working vocal cord to vibrate off the paralyzed left one. Now I can drive, which supports my desire for independence. With each healing milestone I thank God and feel that Somebody up there loves me.

It has not all been bad. During that first year after surgery I was given the gift of time for those things I'd often wanted to do but neglected—like reading the Bible. I found biblical roots for much of what I believed and wrote about. That amazed me. I was encouraged by the faith of evangelists on TV. They gave me hope for healing. I took time to listen to different teachers on cassette tapes and meditate on their words. I saw anew how I had been guided by a higher power all along. I prayed and talked to God many hours each day. I rediscovered my Jewish roots and with them a renewed desire to love and serve humanity.

There were moments of great happiness. My husband, my sister, and my children stood by me. Realizing the depth of their love was a great gift. The love and care I received from family, friends, and even strangers was incredible. One dear friend fasted for me the day of my surgery. Many people prayed for me, and I felt their love in the darkest times. Before the surgery, I called some telephone prayer lines and asked for prayers, something which I still do. With my family and my personal relationship with God, I felt safe and protected, believing I would make it through.

Though I had periods of feeling sorry for myself, I also saw how blessed I was by what I could do easily, like tying my shoes. The hospital was full of people who were worse off than me. I was in tough straits, but at least my prognosis was hopeful. As the old adage goes, "I felt sorry for myself because I had no shoes—and then I met a man who had no feet." The end result of the whole process is that I am tougher now, more at peace and faith-filled. Compared to the hell I was in right after surgery, I'm in heaven now.

Personal growth is always a challenge. My circumstances gave me the opportunity to overcome frustration and release fear, exercise faith, learn trust and patience, and surrender control to a wise and loving higher power. Progress seemed so slight at first. But my husband told me ages ago, "The strength of your growth will be your belief without proof." Faith is indeed belief without proof. During the times when life didn't seem worth living, I was strengthened by that seed of faith planted within me. Though I now have strong faith, I still look for proof. And proof comes in bits and pieces, with each subtle change in me. But the faith came first.

Throughout my healing I used the tools that I describe in this book. For example, visualization: Each time a therapist taught me some new maneuver, like how to stand up, I practiced it in my mind as well as with my body. My physical therapy went smoothly and I gained strength and ability quickly.

The healing of the nervous system continues for years and my prognosis remains excellent. However, in the natural or physical world, no health care professional will guarantee how much healing will occur. But in the spiritual, metaphysical, supernatural world, God through His word promises me healing. Since we tend to get what we believe, I live on those words, believing in my eventual full recovery. Please believe and be in agreement with me. The Spiritual Law of Agreement, through our shared belief focused on a goal, activates a tremendous amount of healing power.

Getting sick, paralyzed, deaf, and afraid enabled me to write this book from a point of deep personal understanding. I am now allowing my healing and release from fear to joy, from disability to enabledness, from imperfection to perfection, from burden to unconditional love and service. I thank God and my doctors for saving me from the tumor. It really was a miracle. This book—about the kinds of thoughts, images, and words which can help us to heal—is part of my thanks.

Self-Help Experience #1
Practice in Self-Awareness Makes Perfect

Purpose: This exercise will add to your self-knowledge by helping you to recognize your emotions and their effect on you physically. Read through all the instructions first and then follow them with your eyes closed. Have a pen and paper ready to make notes after the exercise. Find a quiet place where you will not be disturbed for a few minutes. Relax and then begin.

Can you recall a time when you realized you were really unhappy about a situation? Perhaps you didn't want to face that unhappiness. Perhaps you thought that admitting you were angry, hurt, or sad would lead you into trouble, letting you feel or do something that you didn't want to feel or do. When you recognize and release those emotions, the body becomes healthier and more relaxed. When you are ill, you are guided into right action by observing your symptoms as metaphors. Be prepared for those times by practicing observing what you are experiencing right now. Don't judge—just observe yourself. In other words, at least during this exercise, accept your feelings. Don't put yourself down for what you are feeling.

Use this technique of *witnessing yourself* when you feel physical or emotional pain, or tension. You can put the following instructions on a tape recorder to play back to yourself or have a friend read them to you. Be sure to pause, leaving some quiet time after reading or recording each instruction.

Instructions

1. Take a comfortable position either sitting or lying down. Relax.

2. Allow your attention to rest or focus on different parts of your body—from your toes to the top of your head.

3. Describe to yourself what you are feeling physically and emotionally at this very moment.

4. Notice the thoughts you are thinking.

5. Recall an unhappy incident and repeat steps 2–4. Notice if there is a change in your thoughts and feelings from the way you felt before recalling the unhappy incident. Pause for a few minutes.

6. Stop thinking about the unhappy memory. Release it completely. Now recall a different situation, one that made you angry. Repeat steps 2–4. Become aware of any change in your thoughts and feelings. Pause for a few moments.

7. Stop thinking about the angry memory. Think about something else.

8. Finally, recall a happy time and repeat the first four steps. Again notice any change in your thoughts and feelings. Pause.

9. Smile to yourself.

10. Open your eyes and review what you've learned about yourself, your emotions and your body during this witnessing experience. It can help if you write down what you've learned though this is not necessary to the success of the exercise.

Every so often during the day, check your body for tension. For example, check your hands. Are they clenched or open? How about your mouth—are you gritting your teeth? Are you smiling? Frequent daily body checks will enhance self-awareness. Practice does make perfect.

A primary benefit of this exercise is that you will be more aware of your own feelings and empowered to identify your typical responses to those feelings. This awareness gives you the *freedom to choose your future actions, rather than the automatic knee-jerk reactions typical of many people.* You are not quite as much at the mercy of your emotions if you are aware of their effects on you.

Which came first,
the chicken or the egg?
He pined away and died of grief

Perspectives on Healing

1

Long ago people recognized the interconnectedness of mind, body, and spirit and its relationship to health. For centuries it was taken for granted that people could "die of grief," that unrequited love could cause a person to "pine away," that fear could make one "deathly afraid," that anger could cause illness. Then, in the nineteenth century, the germ theory implicated bacteria in infection, which had been responsible for much illness and death throughout the centuries. Unfortunately, the discovery of the role of germs in causing disease impeded the previous understanding of the link between emotions and health.

Today medicine is adept at eliminating the effects of bacteria and some viruses through vaccination, improved sanitation, and powerful drugs. Yet drugs do not heal or regrow damaged tissue. Furthermore, suppression of symptoms at times leads to problems of cell degeneration—problems often more serious than the original infection.

Even so, mainstream medical practitioners (with the exception of psychiatrists) still largely ignore the role of the mind and emotions in causing and healing disease.

Conventional medicine focuses on the suppression or alteration of symptoms such as unwanted physical sensations. Traditional doctors use drugs and surgery to suppress or remove symptoms. Yet in many cases different symptoms replace the original ones. Removing symptoms doesn't necessarily lead to healing or a cure.

Why do some people suffer illnesses when exposed to viruses and bacteria while others, exposed to the same microorganisms, remain healthy? Even with the idea that fatigue, weakness, and prior illnesses lower one's resistance to infection, the germ theory provides only a partial explanation of illness. Traditionally, each symptom or set of symptoms is considered a separate disease entity, ignoring the emotional connections linking the new set of symptoms to a previous disease.

Holistic Medicine

Today, holistic medicine helps heal the patient by providing a *whole* viewpoint. It views the patient from the total perspective of body, mind, and spirit. Each of these is an aspect of being human and no part can be eliminated if full healing is to occur. Holistic medical practice includes orthodox medical approaches to each of these human aspects, as well as alternative therapies. It represents the cooperation of traditional and non-traditional approaches. This is what Dr. Robert Atkins calls "complementary medicine" in his book *Dr. Atkins' Health Revolution*. Holistic medicine increasingly understands the role language plays in translating thoughts and emotions into physical conditions.

Holistic medicine doesn't ignore bacteria, viruses, or any physical causes of disease. Rather, this approach recognizes many causal factors, including some traditional ones like heredity and environment. These causal factors are integrated with the knowledge of the power of the mind and emotions to predispose us to health or illness.

The mind's power lies in its ability to think, reason, remember, and create images. With our conscious awareness, we choose the images and thoughts we want to dwell on. Some images support well-being while others encourage the illness and suffering that continue to ravage humanity. Today many more doctors accept the idea that emotions affect the body. But they don't really know how or why.

A good doctor knows that what you tell yourself about what happens to you makes a very deep impression. How you feel about your current and past life circumstances, including what you tell yourself about them, can add stress to your life or make the stress less damaging. Holistic healing professionals take time to talk to their patients, to *really listen* to their ideas, to explore the emotional component of any symptoms the patient is experiencing. A truly holistic doctor understands that talking things out helps to prevent and/or relieve the physical symptoms related to an emotional experience.

Dr. Marvin Schweitzer, a key member of my personal team of health helpers, is a Naturopathic Doctor or N.D. practicing in Norwalk, Connecticut. A naturopath has years of training similar to a Medical Doctor, but instead of learning about and using drugs, naturopaths learn more about natural things like food and herbs—nature's botanical medicines. Schweitzer's practice is structured in a way that allows him *time* to really get to know his patients. He told me, "I can't understand why everyone doesn't practice this way. It's so rewarding.

"A person's quality of life does not depend solely on his current health status but also on the attitude towards the illness—towards whatever is going on. Two people can have the identical diagnosis, yet one person's life is a living hell, while the other person's life is filled with happiness. When a person is living fully and with joy—no matter what the circumstances—that opens my heart. That person inspires me and becomes my teacher."

Healing Through Cleansing

Pollution can be seen as a common factor in most illnesses—pollution of the body with toxic wastes and pollution of the mind with negative thoughts. Both may lead to emotions like depression, anger, resentment, and so on. *Digestive* pollution comes from eating the wrong foods or overeating in general. *Environmental* pollution puts stress on the physical body and reduces its resistance. *Language* pollution comes from negative words and fearful thoughts that create harmful stress. All three pollutions are usually present in disease. Everything that isn't in harmony with the body pollutes it. *We get well by releasing our pollution.*

We cleanse ourselves of most digestive and environmental pollutants through rest, fever, and fasting. After ridding the body of infectious or toxic material, the next step is to alter the underlying thought patterns and emotional stresses that allow germs to take root. Mental and emotional fasting—thinking thoughts that won't invite germs in—helps the body to remain free of illness and disease.

If you give a body a chance, it has the means to destroy illness-causing agents. The heat of a fever activates the antibodies in the blood and lymph system to stop germs. Symptoms like fever, swelling, and discharge may be the very means the body uses to heal itself. Suppressing these symptoms may stop the deeper healing process. On the other hand, listening to the message of disease and then acting appropriately gives the body a chance to heal itself by using its own defensive systems. This kind of self-healing often strengthens the body's future resistance to disease.

At the present time we are adept at removing the symptoms of illness using medicines and surgery. But few people know how to use the mind as a tool for healing the physical body. The average person can't even conceive that he might cause himself illness or that he can "uncause" that illness by changing destructive thought patterns and altering self-damaging behaviors. These are not skills we are generally taught. Yet using them we can release the mind's language pollution.

Many people feel more comfortable in the role of victim of disease. They want a doctor to do something to make them better. The idea of taking a drug to cure a disease seems simpler to accept than the idea of self-healing. And it may be easier for most people. But as researchers recognize the increasingly toxic side effects of many drugs, it is prudent to seek other less intrusive, more natural, and often less costly healing techniques. A doctor's responsibility is to use his training to help you to help yourself. But final responsibility for your health rests with you. You decide whether to use what's available or not.

Psychosomatics

At the turn of the century, Sir William Osler—a medical giant—anticipated psychosomatic medicine by declaring, "The care of tuberculosis depends more on what the patient has in his head than what he has in his chest."

Psychosomatic (both physiological and psychological) medicine does recognize the role of mind and emotions in disease. But when psychosomatic medicine was first popularized, many people perceived the label "psychosomatic illness" as derogatory. "Psychosomatic" came to mean "all in the mind" or unreal. It became jargon for "hypochondriac." It implied that the patient was not really feeling the symptoms but only making them up. Some people even thought they were crazy when told that what they felt was not real. To many people, any reference to "mind" in an illness meant "crazy." "It's all in your mind" was a diagnosis to be feared.

The reality of the matter is that disease is a *product of the mind,* and not "all in the mind." The mental and emotional causes of disease produce real physical effects. When you are feeling ill, you are actually *feeling* ill no matter what the cause.

Old-fashioned psychosomatic medicine often seemed to imply that some illnesses were real and others were not. "Real" illness implied physical or organic change or damage. Thus, "not real" illness—meaning non-physical—was *all* in your mind. Holistic medicine is rapidly changing that idea by recognizing that you do actually feel within your body sensations that result from an event in your mind.

Sometimes your body reacts and you are not aware of any physical sensations. Hypertension (high blood pressure) often reflects this truth. You have a physical reaction to emotional pressures. You learn about your bodily reaction only after having a blood pressure reading.

Any emotion from laughter to sadness to fear provokes a physiological response. There is no such thing as *all in your mind.* There is the mental component of your feelings and the physical reaction of your body.

Joan Borysenko has a Ph.D. from Harvard Medical School in cellular biology. She co-founded the mind/body clinic at Beth

Israel Hospital in Boston. Dr. Borysenko's main research interest is the effect of mind on immunity. In her book *Minding the Body, Mending the Mind,* writing about neuropeptides (hormonal messengers) she says, "there is a rich and intricate two-way communication system linking the mind, the immune system, and potentially all other systems, a pathway through which our emotions—our hopes and fears—can affect the body's ability to defend itself."[1]

"In laboratory experiments, we've learned that stress whether acute or chronic, releases a whole array of hormones that provide quick energy. Two of these hormones—adrenalin and cortisol—are also potent inhibitors of the immune system."[2]

In one study that Dr. Borysenko conducted with her husband, immunologist Dr. Myrin Borysenko, Dr. Bruce Crary, and Dr. Herbert Benson, volunteers were injected with a tiny dose of adrenalin—enough to produce the same reaction in you if someone yelled "Boo." Blood tests revealed an immediate decline in lymphocytes, the helper cells that augment the response of the immune system. This shows the immediate effect that fear has on the body at a cellular level.

In another study, this one using dental students, Borysenko, her husband, and other colleagues discovered "that the stress of examination periods reduced the level of a particular antibody in saliva, an antibody that is part of the first line of defense against colds. Exam time is typically when students are most likely to catch colds."[3] After psychological testing of their subjects, they further concluded that students with a more easygoing attitude showed *less* of a drop in antibodies than the other students. Borysenko noted studies by doctors at Ohio State confirm that exam stress reduces the effectiveness of lymphocyte cells whose function is the destruction of virus-infected and cancerous cells.

Borysenko writes, "Disease, however, is rarely a simple matter of isolated cause and effect. While stress and helplessness can depress immune function, clearly we don't get sick each time we're stressed. It's far more reasonable to consider stress as one of many factors that may tip the balance toward illness."

Norman Cousins, well-known editor and author of *Anatomy of an Illness* tells how he used laughter to help cure a stress-produced "incurable" collagen disease. By laughing heartily at movies of his favorite comedians, he was able to get pain-free, drug-free sleep and a boost toward full recovery. Science has since learned that love, laughter ("internal jogging" as Cousins calls it), and other positive emotions and actions rally the body's natural defenses against stress, pain, and disease. Laughing at jokes, at the human condition, and at yourself can help you live longer and happier.

Recognizing that the will to live, the capacity for joy, and self-confidence are important components of total health care, not alternatives to orthodox medicine, Cousins recently wrote, "The wise physician favors a spirit of responsible participation by the patients in a total strategy of medical care...There has been enough replication of research involving controlled studies to point to a presiding fact; namely the physician has a prime resource at his disposal in the form of the patient's own apothecary, especially when combined with the prescription pad."[4]

Your thoughts, fears, and emotions often stimulate detectable physical conditions, though you are almost never conscious of this link or in conscious control of it. But the implications of this discovery are stunning: *if you make disease happen, you also have the power to change it, even to get rid of it*. Disease often forces people to alter negative thoughts, useless behaviors, and ill feelings. Through the power of your *mind*, you control the *matter* that is your body. From the poly-pharmacy of more than fifty hormones produced in your brain which stimulate the various organs of your body, your mind does influence matter. Anything that interferes with the production and dispersal of these hormones has an impact on your body.

Linguistic Dualism

Just as *nose* and *thumb* refer to different parts of one body, *mind* and *body* refer to different aspects of the same whole. Every emotion you feel and every thought you think is also a physical event. Though mind and body are inseparable, dictionaries often define words such as "mind" and "body," "mental" and "physical," and "psychic" and "somatic" as antonyms or opposites. Actually they are functionally inseparable.

Dr. David Graham of the University of Wisconsin Medical School calls mind-versus-body terminology *linguistic dualism.* "The convenience of the separation exists, but it is important to remember that this is nothing more than a linguistic convenience. It is in direct opposition to the way you actually work."[5] Just as the water and the land overlap at the shore, the body and mind have many points of intersection. Rivers and streams flow above and below ground until they finally merge and find full expression in the sea. So too, emotions and thoughts often express themselves in the physical body.

"Psychological" and "physical" and their synonyms refer to *different ways of talking about the same event.* Acne for example, has a physical component—reddening of the skin, eruptions containing toxic material and painful sensations. Depending on the severity of the condition, emotions such as shame or embarrassment may result. People with this condition often think their face looks ugly and fear others will reject them. Acne has a psychological component as well: it can *cause* depression or *result from* depression.

Others with acne may react in a very different way. They may not mind their condition, believing acne is a way for the body to rid itself of wastes through the skin. Still others believe acne is an inevitable result of adolescence that will pass. Thus there are different perspectives from which to view a disease process, including physical and psychological. The event "acne" is a multi-dimensional experience.

The medical profession has encouraged the mind/body division by often ignoring the mind when treating physical symptoms. It unnaturally divided the body into parts and organs, implicitly undermining the reality that every part of the body, every organ, affects every other. The medical profession in general, and medical specialists in their fields, have brought us enormous benefits, and their contribution should not be downplayed. But specialists are often limited because they see their patients as series of parts to be healed rather than as whole human beings. By forgetting about the body's mental and emotional connections, they rarely recognize the creative role of the mind in all physical disease.

When we began to define the parts of the body by their functions—the heart is just a pump, the stomach is a sack, hearing is the result of some bones vibrating in the head, muscles are pulleys—we moved away from understanding man as greater than the sum of his parts, and ceased understanding the wholeness of man at all. It's important to understand how each part works, but something valuable gets lost in the process.

Ronald J. Glasser, M.D., in *The Body Is The Hero* wrote, "we know, even if our surgeons and internists don't, that we are connected with our bodies, that the catch in our breath when we are startled, the tension in our guts when we're worried, the exhaustion we feel from our anxiety are as much a part of our illnesses as are the bacteria, viruses and auto-antibodies which attack us, and can in fact be just as debilitating and just as deadly."[6] To fully cure anyone of anything, it's important to treat the whole patient, mind and emotions as well as body.

Some cultures continue to recognize that all parts of the human are involved in the disease process. Medicine men and shamans treat both mind and body. Through potions and incantations they work on the physical and spiritual levels. The use of these rituals opens the mind to the reality that healing will occur, releasing negativity. Medicine men and some present-day healers recognize that a mind open to the possibility of healing allows the process to begin and move more easily to completion.

Open Mind, Whole Mind

When cancer was viewed as a sure death sentence, the patient often gave up hope. Today this former certainty has changed. Cancer patients have hope. Now AIDS is considered hopeless by almost everyone, despite growing evidence to the contrary. Carolyn Reuben recently wrote in *East West Journal* that many AIDS patients remain in remission, living years beyond the expectations of their doctors. But they rarely talk about it because, says Reuben, "the belief system is so strong in our society that they will die. By saying you're in remission everybody who doesn't believe it's possible and thinks it's only temporary and you will die projects the thought form at you. You have to be a really strong individual."[7]

Wider knowledge about AIDS patients who survive longer than expected may save lives by giving other AIDS patients hope. Many cancer patients have strengthened their immune systems by using techniques such as visualization and meditation. It is not unreasonable to assume that AIDS patients can help themselves survive, given the right incentive: belief that survival is possible.

Recently, several AIDS patients who have survived years longer than expected appeared on television. All of them "changed their minds" as part of their healing process. One woman who appeared on "The Phil Donohue Show" on June 20, 1989 said that three years ago she had ARC—AIDS Related Complex. Today she is well, with no signs of disease; she tests free of the AIDS virus. Finally, the March 1989 edition of *Brain/Mind Bulletin* had an article about a recently held AIDS symposium at which ten long-term AIDS survivors spoke on a panel. Death from AIDS is not inevitable. There is always hope.

Words and thoughts alone don't cause disease. But thoughts affect us by triggering responses in the body which lead to chemical, hormonal, neurological, and muscular changes. Biofeedback instruments demonstrate the effect of thoughts and emotions on the body, for instance proving that muscles are activated when we think about anything involving action. Among the many biofeedback tools that can help us recognize how our body is behaving are *thermometers,* which measure body temperature; *sphygmomanometers,* which measure blood pressure; and *electromyography (EMG),* which measures electric currents associated with muscular action and hence body relaxation. A beeper on the EMG alerts the subject when certain muscles become too tense. Used in re-training body responses, the EMG is a powerful tool for releasing stress and increasing self-knowledge.

Until I studied biofeedback I never realized how tense I had been when having my blood pressure taken. Trying to relax, I often became more tense. I would shut my eyes and hold my breath, leading to increased body tension. This is obvious to me now, but I was less conscious at the time, and thought I was relaxing. To train me, a psychologist guided me through Progressive Muscle Relaxation (a technique explained at the end of this chapter). When

I was successful in turning off the beeper, the EMG confirmed objectively the depth of relaxation I subjectively felt.

Thought Affects Physiology

Physicist and psychologist Buryl Payne, Ph.D., writes:

> We know that thoughts generated in the brain activate hormone secretions and stimulate other nerve centers within the body. Thoughts, coded as neural impulses, travel along nerve axons, activating muscles and glands similar to the manner in which telephone messages travel over wires in the form of electrical signals. Experiments with the GSR, a biofeedback instrument, attached to fingers or toes clearly demonstrate that mental activity reaches into the extremities of the body.
>
> With sensitive EMG instruments, we can show that muscles are activated when we think about anything involving action or emotion, even though there may be no visible movement. Although we do not know how thoughts are generated in the brain, it seems clear that once present, thoughts are amplified by the brain and turned into actions. Every thought we think influences millions of atoms, molecules, and cells throughout the body. Besides this straightforward effect on the physical body, we know from general principles of physics that any acceleration of electrons produces some electromagnetic radiation."[8]

There is ample documentation in the medical literature of the effects of strong emotion on the human body. Strong emotions are triggered by moving events or experiences. Emotions are real, primal, instinctive—raw feelings triggered by events and experiences and sometimes the experience of a thought. But usually thoughts are our attempt to give meaning to our emotions. The quality of our thoughts determines how well we cope with emotional experiences and influences whether we feel well or dis-eased. People can literally die after being "scared to death."

Norman Cousins cites a study, reported by George Engel, of people who died in response to shattering news. In the study 27 percent of the people who died suddenly from emotional shock had been confronted with "grave" personal danger. Engel in turn quoted another study by J.C. Barker, which described forty-two cases of people who died abruptly after being frightened. Cousins comments, "Folklore and medical science come together in accepting the reality of sudden death through emotional causes. Folklore makes note of the fact; medical science understands what happens inside the body to bring it about."[9] Apparently sudden emotional shock may touch off a dangerously rapid and erratic heartbeat, technically known as fibrillation. Cousins's theme is that "nothing is more essential in the treatment of serious disease than liberating the patient from panic and foreboding."[10]

Grief, too, is a potent emotional force. A person can literally "die of a broken heart." James J. Lynch, Scientific Director of the Psychosomatic Clinics at the University of Maryland School of Medicine has this to say about the effects of human companionship on health: "the 'broken heart' is not just a poetic image for loneliness and despair—it is a medical reality. In our fragmented society, the lack of human companionship—chronic loneliness and social isolation as well as the sudden loss of loved ones—is one of the leading causes of premature death. And while lack of human companionship is related to virtually every major disease from cancer and tuberculosis to mental illness, the link is particularly marked in the case of heart disease, the nation's leading killer. Every year millions die, quite literally, of a broken or lonely heart."[11]

Strong emotions can produce the physiological changes that allow disease conditions to flourish. These strong emotions are often triggered by thoughts. Psychiatrist Andrew Weil, speaking on "The Phil Donohue Show" in June of 1987 said, "Disordered thinking can produce disordered brain chemistry." By noticing such harmful thoughts as "I am sick and tired of that," or even "I am scared to death" you will begin to recognize your own connections between language and disease. With this increased awareness you can begin to eliminate those thoughts and *feel* for yourself if there is a change in your level of well-being.

Paul Pearsall in his book *Superimmunity* reports on the results of Drs. Elmer and Alyce Green's examination of four hundred cases of spontaneous remissions in cancer patients. He defines spontaneous remission as "all of a sudden the disease went away and we have no idea why, and we didn't seem to do anything to make it go away based on our treatment." The Greens "found only one factor common to each case they examined. All these people had changed their attitude prior to the remission and, in some way, had found hope and become more positive in their approach to the disease."[12]

Pearsall writes, "It puzzles me that physicians sometimes forget that the bombardment of the system with deadly chemicals against cancer is also related to how we feel and that spontaneous remissions occur during these treatment regimens as well. Studies on the successes of radiation and chemotherapy seldom report on changes in the belief systems and attitudes of the patients receiving the treatment. It seems equally plausible that people's belief systems change when an encouraging, trusted doctor, in this case serving in the role of shaman or healer, administers a magic elixir in the form of strong chemicals or buzzing machines that alter not only cell biology but personal psychology."

As information about the power of thoughts becomes more widespread, increased research takes place into the role of mind in healing. Perhaps the cure for cancer and AIDS will be found in patients' beliefs as much as in more potent drugs. The holistic approach to healing including psychological approaches and medical technology seems the wisest course for any seriously ill patient. The search for medicines that assist in healing should continue. And the search for newer, more powerful mental technology should expand. Then the software called mind can be brought into play to expand the potential of the hardware called body.

Self-Help Experience #2
Progressive Muscle Relaxation

Purpose: To help you to be more in touch with the feel of different parts of your body; to assist you in relaxing your body

During biofeedback training I realized that I didn't know how to tense certain parts of my body, because I often couldn't differentiate a tense muscle from a relaxed one. Those muscles weren't initially responsive to my conscious control. Chronically tense or contracted muscles reveal a habitual response pattern in one's life—usually below one's conscious level of awareness. Practice in tensing and releasing ultimately leads to increased awareness and a finely-tuned ability to release tension more easily.

Progressive muscle relaxation is an exercise to de-stress and relax your body. It involves clenching and releasing muscles in different parts of the body. Your eyes may be open or shut, though focusing within is easier with eyes shut.

Instructions

1. Begin by getting into a relaxed position, either lying down or sitting in a comfortable chair.

2. Clench your right hand into a fist.

3. Observe the sensations in your hand, arm, shoulder, or elsewhere in your body, for a few seconds.

4. Release your fist by opening your hand and relaxing.

5. Notice the differences in sensation between the clenched and the released state.

6. Do this process several times.

7. Tighten your stomach muscles. Observe your physical sensations in your stomach and in the rest of your body

8. Relax your stomach muscles and notice how you feel. Tighten and relax a few times.

9. Contract your buttocks. Notice how this feels. Then release the tightened buttocks muscles and observe how you feel.

10. Contract the muscles of your head including the eyes, the forehead, your cheeks, and chin. How does each one feel? Relax the muscles and observe the differences in feeling.

As you get adept at this clenching and releasing process, you can isolate any area you wish to work on. Pay special attention to the head, neck, and stomach. It takes about twenty minutes per session until you master the process. At the end of each practice session, stop actively tensing. Then, just *imagine* your fist being clenched. Don't do it. Just *think* it. Notice if you are still relaxed. After several weeks of performing this process, you will feel less tense. You may discover *where* in your body you are holding tension. In places where you are chronically tense, you may not be aware of the muscles until you begin to release the tension.

Self-Help Experience #3
The Pendulum

Purpose: To observe a thought affecting your body

You can test the effects of your thoughts on your body by trying the following experiment. Use a necklace with a pendant or tie a weight (like a ring) on a piece of string in order to create a pendulum. Sit in a relaxed position, with the elbow of the arm that is holding the pendulum resting on a table. Think about the pendulum moving, but don't make it move by moving your arm. Tell yourself that you *will* the pendulum to move. You may suggest the direction (sideways, front–to–back, or diagonally) or not. Holding the pendulum without trying to move it in any way, allow the pendulum to move by itself.

You can keep your eyes closed until you seem to feel the pendulum moving—then you can peek. You will be amazed how your thoughts cause the pendulum to swing without you moving your hand. Some minute neuromuscular mechanism controlled subconsciously is probably at work, something so subtle that most of us are not aware of it.

Self-Help Experience #4
Developing Inner Peace and Harmonizing Your Thoughts

Purpose: To determine how and to what degree your thoughts affect you emotionally and physically. This exercise provides practice in observing and releasing unwanted thoughts and letting go of obsessions.

Notice what types of thoughts improve your sense of well-being and what circumstances surround those thoughts. The average person has thousands of thoughts a day—some we call positive: hopes, dreams, memories of happy times, loving feelings, and so on; some we call negative: worries, jealousies, insecurities, angers, cravings for forbidden things.

Some people believe we need to accept negative thoughts. In a sense that's true. We can learn much about ourselves from our so-called negative thoughts. But we must also be able to let them go. Positive and negative are based on our own mental judgments.

Sometimes we get stuck in thinking about an experience. We dwell on it so much that we can't get on with life. To restore harmony within, you must learn to "get off it," to change the place where your mind is dwelling. *You can choose what to think.* If an unwanted thought spontaneously arises, you can rid yourself of that thought by replacing it with another thought of your choice. *The mind can only think one complete thought at a time.* After a while it will become second nature for you to replace your unwanted negative thoughts with desirable positive ones.

Instructions

1. For the next few days, frequently throughout the day, stop what you are doing and observe what you are thinking. Observe yourself objectively. Notice if your thoughts are helpful or unhelpful. Label them positive or negative.

2. When an unwanted thought arises and you want to release it and restore harmony in your mind, pause in what you are doing.

3. Take slow deep breaths, flushing your system with oxygen to lower your level of anxiety. Pay attention to your breath. You will soon reach a relaxed, helpful state called the *alpha* state, when your brain waves shift from an alert beta rhythm to a relaxed alpha rhythm.

4. Think about a pleasant scene: a mountain lake, a beach, any favored place of relaxation, or think about some upcoming event which you are looking forward to.

5. Practice this technique often throughout the day until you notice the number of upsetting thoughts decrease.

How We Talk
About Disease

2

J ames Lance, in the book *Headache: Understanding Alleviation,* provides us with a poignant example of the body's response to words. "The dramatic term whiplash injury conjures up a vision of the patient's neck being cracked like a whip—imagery more vivid than is usually warranted by the circumstances. The very use of the term may be enough to make the patient retract his neck like a tortoise, causing the neck muscles to contract continuously, a potent cause of headache in its own right."[13]

Names as Symbols Evoke Images

The power of a name lies in its ability to evoke an image. Mention the name of a loved one and a set of feelings, thoughts, and images appear—perhaps many conflicting images. Mention the name of a place and a differ ent set of feelings and thoughts arise. Mention the name of a disease like cancer or acne and still another set of images occur, perhaps accompanied by strong negative feelings. Negative

27

feelings include worries, fears, depressions, jealousies, and hates, among others. Since they teach us about ourselves, they aren't bad. But left untended, these feelings can lead to illness.

The names of things matter because the images they evoke shape our thoughts and feelings, which in turn affect our bodies. As we name a thing we are also, in a sense, causing or creating it. The name reminds us of a previously encoded image that our body can then recreate. Expectation plays a major role. In an obvious example, placing the label "heartbroken" on an emotional response can cause actual physical distress.

We have a tendency to want to name everything that happens to us. To avoid the ambiguity of not knowing and not understanding, we tend to label uncomfortable bodily states. Naming a set of symptoms often brings relief because people assume that knowing the name means something can be done about the illness. The name of a disease is important in planning treatment, so finding the right name *is* necessary. The diagnosis thus leads to treatment to relieve the unwanted condition. However, the name can also evoke unwanted images and expectations. These negatively influence the disease process, stressing an already strained body.

The label "cancer" causes fear in many people—even though the predicted outcome of a bout with cancer continues to improve. Tuberculosis had the same effect in the nineteenth century. Our present "label of death" is the word "AIDS." It invokes terror, because a fatal outcome from this disease is said to be inevitable. When the results of treatment for AIDS improve, as cause and cure are found, the label won't lead to the hopeless feeling that often insures a negative end result. Doctors, who are the purveyors of the name for a set of symptoms, can influence a patient's expectations by presenting the diagnosis in a framework of hope.

Often only some of the symptoms of a particular disease are present at the time that a label is attached to an illness. The patient might then *expect* the missing symptoms to occur. Or, for instance, the physician might ask the patient whether she is experiencing other expected symptoms, presenting a subtle suggestion to the patient's mind.

Paul Pearsall in *Superimmunity* reports making the terrible mistake of asking one of his pregnant counseling patients, "Have you had morning sickness yet?" She responded that she was feeling just fine, "I can't believe how good the pregnancy is going." The next day she called Pearsall to report spending most of the night experiencing nausea. She concluded, "I really have it now."[14] Pearsall recognized that asking the question was probably stimulus to his client's response.

Expectations often generate the unwanted result. However, in practice, not everyone gets every symptom of a particular disease or condition, just as lots of women, myself included, never experience morning sickness when they are pregnant. On the contrary, give a person the proper physical, mental, and emotional support and the body can cure just about any disease.

The Advent of the Sinus Headache

When a particular set of feelings and behaviors—"symptoms"—are grouped together and named, a new disease emerges. The identification of the disease called AIDS led to the research that will eventually define the actions necessary to cure it. But sometimes naming a set of symptoms generates new victims.

In communication theory, the Sapir-Whorf hypothesis states: When you have a name for something, you are much more likely to perceive it. The classic example is that of the Eskimos. They have dozens of words for different kinds of snow, and they *see* all those different kinds. Those of us who live in more temperate climates have only one word for snow, with a few variations, so that one kind of snow is all we perceive. John Bear, Ph.D., told me the following story, which illustrates the above effect:

> The notion that you feel, experience, and suffer from things for which you have words became clear to me in the early 60s. At a big New York advertising agency, I met a man famous in the annals of advertising because he had invented a disease. You see, when a new drug comes along, it requires years of testing before the Food and Drug Administration approves it. This man's stroke of genius was to take an already approved drug—one that was languishing in sales— and invent a new disease that the drug could help. New diseases do not have to be approved by the FDA!

> The drug in question was Dristan, then a modestly-selling cold and headache remedy. This man invented the name "sinus headache." He named a collection of symptoms which were then recognized as a

new disease. He used language to distinguish this entirely new headache. Actually, people had probably often suffered head pain from sinus distress without knowing why. Now they knew! This advertising genius then wrote a whole series of advertisements presenting Dristan as the only product that could cure a sinus headache. All over America, people suddenly started having sinus headaches in ever increasing numbers, propelling Dristan onto the bestseller list of over-the-counter remedies. Nearly 20 years later, the sinus headache has become a standard ailment which even appears in some medical texts. Such is the power of language in creating disease.

Anorexia and Bulimia

Much attention has recently been focused on the eating disorders called anorexia and bulimia. There were some people engaging in anorexic and bulimic behaviors who didn't know they had a disease until they heard the names and learned what they represented. Long before I knew the word "bulimia," an acquaintance introduced me to the idea of vomiting to control weight—although it never appealed to me personally. Perhaps anorexic and bulimic behaviors seem more prevalent now, because they have been named and publicized.

However, it is possible that many people who aren't sick have been falsely labeled "anorexic." I find myself wondering about several women friends who are very thin. Attaching labels to people is dangerous since people have a tendency to become what we expect of them. On the other hand, perhaps the fear of anorexia will help release some people addicted to the idea that only thin is beautiful.

Does the name of a disease, like "sinus headache" or "anorexia" help people to feel less alone by naming the symptoms they are experiencing and the behaviors they are engaged in? Does the name encourage them to seek treatment? Or does the name plant an idea in their consciousness, encouraging some people to adopt the behaviors and develop the symptoms? Which comes first, the name or the disease?

We are familiar with the copycat crime syndrome in which unusual crimes, when reported in the media, cause rashes of similar crimes. In the same way there may be a copycat disease syndrome. A classic example of this occurred several years ago in Los

Angeles. During a game at Monterey Park Football Stadium several people began experiencing symptoms of food poisoning. Soft drinks from a particular machine were the suspected cause. An announcement was broadcast over the stadium public address system warning patrons that drinks from such a machine could cause severe nausea and other symptoms. Soon, hundreds of people began exhibiting similar symptoms of food poisoning. Many were even hospitalized for observation. Shortly thereafter, it was announced that the soft drink machine was not involved in the food poisoning. Immediately people's symptoms began to clear.

People tend to imitate the behavior of others. When they hear of certain behaviors, this at least implants the idea that such behaviors are possible, a possibility that might never have otherwise occurred to them. This could be significant in relation to anxiety diseases like phobias. Some people develop phobias after hearing about them. The same could be said about any of the compulsive disease disorders.

On the other hand, people often seek treatment after hearing about such a disease. Talk shows hosts like Oprah, Donohue, Geraldo, and Sally Jessy Raphael often have informational shows about what can best be described as medical oddities. These less well-known conditions, such as self-mutilation, compulsive disorder syndrome, or ultra-severe obesity, may afflict hundreds of viewers. They first hear about possible treatments during these talk shows. Sometimes, these people hadn't even realized they were suffering from a real disease that has a cure rate from a defined treatment plan. Here, information is power.

When you describe an action, you can reinforce the idea of engaging in that action. Research into the lives of husbands of pregnant women indicates that some husbands exhibit many of the sensations and behaviors associated with pregnancy, like food cravings and morning sickness. Medical students are known to often exhibit the symptoms of diseases they are studying. These imitations may not be common, but they do occur. Ideas have power.

While diagnosing and naming a disease can be very useful in the healing process, some of the negative effects of naming are less obvious. Names are always nouns. Naming a disease as a noun reinforces the idea that anorexia, arthritis, cancer, heart attack, or even strep throat and whiplash, are things that "just happen to us" and which we cannot control or be responsible for. This use of language reinforces a view of ourselves as victims of the events of our lives. Now we have a particular event which we call a "disease," and we have given it a name. Such language diminishes our feeling of being in control of our lives. Feeling a lack of control has itself been linked to the progress of disease.

Hypertension—high blood pressure—is a disease that seems to be related to feelings of powerlessness. John Sommers-Flanagan of the University of Montana and Roger Greenberg of the State University of New York reviewed forty-eight empirical studies from the past decade which link high blood pressure with various psychological factors. They found evidence of three primary psychological characteristics of hypertensives:

1. Anger/hostility.
2. Difficulty with interpersonal contact and communication.
3. Frequent use of denial and self-repression.

Current treatment for hypertension typically includes drugs, exercise, and diet. As a result of their research, Sommers-Flanagan and Greenberg recommend that psychological approaches be used more often to supplement or even replace traditional medical solutions. Greenberg said, "We felt that the part personality plays has been increasingly undervalued. There seems to have been a trend toward regarding many disorders as exclusively biological. We think an integrated approach is necessary."[15] Psychosocial intervention could enhance the ability of hypertension patients to control the physical effects of their tension-provoking experiences by reducing anxiety and increasing coping skills.

Disease as a Form of Human Behavior

Labeling a person an "alcoholic" or a "drug addict" can be either positive or negative: positive if it helps the person take actions that move her away from that illness; negative if the person feels and continues to act like a victim, stuck forever with a diseased behavior. The label can also create an image in the mind of others which may reinforce the victim's unwanted behavior patterns. The expectations of others can influence our thoughts, our actions and our negative behaviors.

The old adage, "Sticks and stones can break my bones, but names can never harm me" is incorrect. Call someone stupid or lazy and the label can stick, becoming a self-fulfilling prophecy. See someone as an alcoholic or a sugar junkie and you might be feeding their disease. However, you might also be identifying what's wrong with them, leading them to seek help.

In the ongoing, ever-changing drama of health, *psyche* (the mind and emotions) and *soma* (the body) engage in a variety of behaviors. We give meaning to the behaviors, such as good or bad, positive or negative, healthy or sick, well or diseased. We often give the behavior the name of a specific disease. But *disease is a human behavioral process, not just a specific entity with a label and a definition*. The label is merely a convenient way to describe a set of symptoms the ill person experiences. I might hyphenate dis-ease to indicate that when I'm not feeling well, I'm not at ease within myself, that my mind, body, and emotions are out of sync. *Disease is* the opposite of being *at ease*.

The following statements illustrate how we usually talk about sickness:

"I'm getting a cold."

"My child caught chicken pox."

"Jane has measles."

"I had an allergy attack."

All the above examples presuppose disease as something external to us, an invader that is not part of us, something that comes from somewhere else and imposes itself upon us for a time. Something external to us may indeed trigger the disease, but it is *our* body that reacts. These common expressions and labels are useful, often making it unnecessary to describe the symptoms being experienced. But this way of talking also helps us to feel like victims and contributes to our avoiding taking personal responsibility for our health. People who continue to feel like victims often do nothing to help themselves. A responsible person takes action to eliminate the dis-ease.

The grammatical structure of the language of disease suggests that we play no major part in causing an illness. Yet the labels we use to name things have a great deal to do with how we see them. Naming the disease with a noun often conveys the impression that it is *a closed entity rather* than an *on-going process*. When disease is seen as external to ourselves, something we catch or get, we convey the impression that measles, cancer, or acne are conditions over which we have no control. Perhaps we have more control than we know.

If you are obese, saying "I overeat" allows you to recognize yourself as the source of your overweight condition. Once this point of inner control is established, you can choose to change the amount and type of food you eat and your level of physical activity. These changes frequently lead to weight loss and a release from the obesity (a noun) behavior pattern. Recognizing your role in creating dis-ease improves your chances of releasing the disease and returning to good health. Illness comes from how you talk and what you think and feel. You can also change your mind about what is fat and release yourself from any negative self-judgments.

How we think and speak about our lives and ourselves is a key component to living a quality life. The Bible speaks of this in the book of James (Ch 3:3–7):

> If anyone can control his tongue, it proves that he has perfect control over himself in every other way. We can make a large horse turn around and go wherever we want by means of a small bit in his mouth. And a tiny rudder makes a huge ship turn wherever the pilot wants it to go, even though the winds are strong. So also the tongue is a small thing, but what enormous damage it can do. A great forest can be set on fire by one tiny spark. And the tongue is a flame of fire. It is full of wickedness, and poisons every part of the body. And the tongue is set on fire by hell itself, and can turn our whole lives into a blazing flame of destruction and disaster.[16]

You may not want to recognize yourself as the source of your ailments. But until you do, you are not in the driver's seat and cannot begin to *think of yourself as the source of healing as well: you caused it, to some degree, and you can uncause it, to the same degree.*

It is important to accept yourself and learn from past mistakes, rather than cause yourself more dis-ease by feelings of self-hate and guilt. Most health professionals would agree: *Loving yourself is an important component in healing.* A spiritual teacher once told me, "Love yourself fully and then you can love everyone else. Take care of yourself, so you can take care of everyone else." Maybe that's the true meaning of the biblical commandment to love your neighbor as yourself. First, we have to learn how to love ourselves.

Disease is not a thing that happens to you; it is a way of acting out life. You are responsible for everything in your life, whether you believe it or not. When you recognize this truth you will begin to accept that you *are in charge of your health at the subtle level of thoughts as well as the obvious level of actions.* Granted, altering the effects of past thoughts and actions might take quite a while. The process might even seem to be irrevocable if it has gone on too long, but people quite often experience miraculous cures even from socalled "terminal" diseases. Responsibility fosters hope, and that often leads to self-induced healing.

Self-Help Experience #5
Is "Cancer" a Verb?

Purpose: To increase your sense of control over your body

We name diseases with nouns. But since disease is actually a behavioral process we engage in, try using the disease name as a verb. Verbs are process words indicating some action you take. As a semantic exercise, try changing the noun for acne or cancer to a verb.

Say: "I am acne-ing," not "I have acne." "My body is cancer-ing," not "I have cancer." It may be awkward to talk in this way, but which way of talking implies greater personal control?

Use the name of your illness as a verb to indicate that illness as an ongoing process which you act out. See if you don't feel more responsible for what ails you. *Being responsible does not mean blaming yourself.* Being responsible does mean accepting yourself and then doing what's appropriate to help yourself—be it taking medicine or acting in new ways.

Self-Help Experience #6
Questions for Patients with Catastrophic Illness

Purpose: To increase the patient's self-knowledge during illness; to discover the patient's basic attitudes toward being healed

The following are key questions to ask oneself or another at the onset or upon diagnosis of a catastrophic illness. The self-knowledge gained from the answers can motivate the patient toward recovery. After much self-reflection, one woman recognized that she broke her leg so she wouldn't have to continue a teaching job in a school she "couldn't stand." She couldn't quit because she was "supporting" her husband in dental school. Instead, she broke her leg skiing. She said, "The broken leg got me out of teaching. Because I wasn't capable of moving fast in the event of a school fire, I had "no choice" but to stop. But the price of the "accident" was heavy. It took six months for my leg to heal and much of that time I was stuck in the house."

Before answering each question, close your eyes, relax, and look deeply within to find the truth. Take time to contemplate each question. Be wary of automatic answers.

1. *How long do you want to live?* Do you love yourself enough to take care of your mind and body? Do you look forward to the future with hope or fear? These questions help you to uncover your will to live and how much control you feel you have in life.

2. *What happened in the year or two before your illness?* List those experiences, both positive and negative, that had a major impact on you. Examples: getting married or divorced, death of a loved one, getting a new job or being fired, starting or losing a business.

3. *What does the illness mean to you?* Do you consider it an automatic death sentence? Some people expect to live, no matter what the odds. Others expect to die no matter what the odds. You are an individual and can beat the odds either way.

4. *Why do you need this illness?* Since sickness often gives people permission to avoid things they really don't want to do, or to do things they wouldn't permit themselves to do, *this is a key question to ask for any illness, major or minor.* People get sick to take time off from their usual ways of behaving. A bout with colds or flu might be avoided if people took more "personal" days off from work, rather than "sickness days." The sickness allows them to escape their "shoulds." "I should do this…be this…feel this way."

Responsibility and Creative Intelligence

3

The guiding light of the body is the mind. Recognizing the connection between language and wellness enables you to expand your control of your health process. The language connection consists of the thoughts, words, imaginings, mental pictures, and emotions that stimulate illness and wellness. By correctly using your language connection diseasing behavior can be healed. Behavior includes actions, lifestyle, thoughts, and spoken words.

The body often expresses itself in symptoms. You may feel like a victim of this body process (disease), since most symptoms (body behaviors) are not consciously induced. Take pimples, for example: you choose to ignore, squeeze, or medicate a pimple, but you don't consciously choose to have one. During a cold, your body secretes mucus, your nose runs, you sneeze and cough. You can choose to blow your nose, but you aren't aware of choosing to have the excess mucus. Something in you, however, is causing the pimple to erupt or the mucus to secrete. With cancer, cell division runs amok, though the conscious part of your mind wouldn't choose cancering behavior.

Who or what is controlling these body behaviors? How does it know what to do? Is it possible to gain some control over this creative process? Can you guide the inner intelligence that controls the automatic functions and behaviors of your body? Can you choose your level of health or illness? To the last question, the answer is "Yes," to a large degree. *Dis-ease is a process over which you can have more control by carefully choosing your thoughts, your words, your attitude, and your actions.* When you are responsible, you have the choice of altering the way that you think, speak, and act in order to change the effects.

We face many choices in the course of a lifetime. We may not always be able to choose our circumstances. But we have freedom to choose *how we feel about* those circumstances. We can choose to be upset, despairing, angry, and envious—or happy, satisfied, and content. We can ignore our feelings or listen to them and learn from them. Free choice means that we realize we have the choice.

Viktor Frankl, M.D., sheds light on the choices we each can make in *Man's Search for Meaning*. This book, a moving account of his incarceration in various Nazi concentration camps, also presents the basic concepts of logotherapy—a psychotherapy he developed and later refined as a result of those harrowing years in the camps. He wrote,

> The experiences of camp life show that man does have a choice of action. There were enough examples, often of a heroic nature, which proved that apathy could be overcome, irritability suppressed. Man *can* preserve a vestige of spiritual freedom, of independence of mind, even in such terrible conditions of psychic and physical stress.
>
> We who lived in concentration camps can remember the men who walked through the huts comforting others, giving away their last piece of bread. They may have been few in number, but they offer sufficient proof that *everything can be taken from a man but one thing: the last of the human freedoms—to choose one's attitude in any given set of circumstances, to choose one's own way.* In the final analysis it becomes clear that the sort of person the prisoner became was the result of an inner decision, and not the result of camp influences alone. Fundamentally therefore, any man can, even under such circumstances, decide what shall become of him—mentally and spiritually.[17]

Dr. Wallace C. Ellerbroek was for many years a prominent California surgeon, psychiatrist, and amateur psycholinguist. After years of informal research and a formal research project using acne patients, he realized that *disease arises not so much out of what happens to us but as a result of how we see things, and the things we tell ourselves.* He once wrote, "It isn't what happens that bugs you, it's the things that you say in your head about what happens that makes all the machinery get messed up, and leads to varieties of disease."[18]

Dr. Ellerbroek tested his theory of disease on a group of thirty-eight acne patients, aged 13 to 46. Acne patients "pick at" their lesions and they frequently feel "picked on" in life. His patients generally interpreted anything they did not like as abuse aimed personally at them. His thesis was that the acne would improve if the "picked on" thought pattern and other contributory behavior could be decreased or eliminated. He treated them with a combination of psychological and psycholinguistic therapy designed to change the patients' thinking so they no longer felt like victims. Based on subjective observations by himself and the patients, the results were excellent. Of the thirty-eight original patients, thirty were judged 80 percent improved within eight weeks. Over a longer period of time, more than half of the patients achieved clear skin. The remainder showed 80–90 percent improvement. Here is how Dr. Ellerbroek explained his results:

> We humans create mental pictures of what we observe in the external world, our version of reality. This evaluation of reality is often inaccurate, due to limitations of our sensory organs and inadequate mechanisms for verifying our perceptions. At any given moment we have a personal idea of how we think the past, present, and future *should be*. Reality can be seen as the way we *want* it to be, the way we *think* it really is, or the way it *actually is*.
>
> When our world seems to match our picture of how we think it should be, we feel good. When humans become aware that their version of reality doesn't match their fantasy of how it should be, they often irrationally and unconsciously demand that reality be changed to match their fantasy. The failure of reality to alter itself to match their fantasy can lead to depression and frustration, the emotions that are the core of illness.

An example of this unrealistic demand is reflected in the negative emotions felt when we think life isn't going our way. Perhaps the weather spoiled a picnic or an employee called in sick and we must do the extra work. In our fantasy-reality these things are not okay occurrences. To the extent that we deny the validity of these events, we will experience the upsetting emotions that in turn often cause illness. Yet what happened has already happened and can't be changed.

Years spent treating patients as a psychiatrist and surgeon convinced me that mental and physical illness are different manifestations of the same disease process: negative thinking. Your brain is patterned by everything that happens throughout your life, even back to the moment you were conceived. So all the years you were, for example, thinking picked-on thoughts, your brain was recording these. Since we all tend to continue doing whatever we do, it becomes obvious that learning a new process of thinking is not an easy or trivial thing to do. I am also convinced, from my years in practice, that effective treatment is attainable.

An example of people attempting to make reality conform to their pictures has recently occurred in China. The Chinese Communist leadership has attempted to cover up the violence committed against their people. Despite the whole world witnessing these events on TV, the leadership still attempted to convince us that what everyone knows happened didn't really happen.

Acceptance of reality is the beginning of taking responsibility for your life. Often you can control events, but just as often you must adapt to circumstances beyond your control. How you adapt—the thoughts you think, the words you speak, and the attitude you take—determines your state of health and your chance of recovery. Thinking and speaking like a victim discourages healing. You change your experience by first recognizing the role your emotions, thoughts, and speech play in inducing disease.

A big part of your role is to envision and believe that healing is possible. Hope helps! Loss of hope is deadly! Your body's innate wisdom knows how to heal itself. But, it can also create the physical symptoms associated with despair, or any other emotional attitude.

Even cases of so-called "terminal" cancer have been reversed. Recently reports have also emerged about long-time survivors of the usually deadly AIDS virus. An Advanced Immune Discoveries Symposium in Los Angeles featured a panel of ten long-term survivors.[19] AIDS patients and some long-term survivors have appeared on several TV talk shows, often bringing messages of hope. One man said he no longer tests positive for AIDS, although he had had several bouts with AIDS symptoms—pneumonia and cancer. A woman in the audience who had been diagnosed with ARC was also now virus free.

Ronald Glasser, M.D. writes, "It is the body that is the hero, not science, not antibiotics...not machines or new devices....The task of the physician today is what it has always been, to help the body do what it has learned so well to do on its own during its unending struggle for survival—to heal itself. It is the body, not medicine, that is the hero."[20]

Your language affects your body both positively and negatively. When you think about situations that make you angry, your blood pressure can rise. Some people get red in the face. Often the heart beats faster and the jaws clench. These physical reactions are caused by thoughts which trigger emotions and vice versa. Emotions trigger more thoughts as you give meaning to what you feel. This vicious, self-reinforcing cycle, if it becomes a habit, will eventually bring itself graphically to your attention as physical symptoms. Happy thoughts promote healing! A smile or a hearty laugh are stress reducers. Pay attention to those thoughts which promote your well-being and those which make you feel rotten.

Obviously how you feel affects your thoughts and words. When you feel head pain you say, "I have a headache." Less obviously, the process also works in reverse: *what you think and say affects how you feel.* Frustrated over work, you might say, "This project is one big headache." Later your head may actually begin to hurt. You meant to express frustration about the difficulty of a project, not invite pain in. However, your body, run by your unconscious mind, might not understand that you are speaking metaphorically. Your unconscious mind can create an unwanted condition in your body by taking your statements quite literally. At the cellular level, the mind does not understand what you really mean. It cannot distinguish fact from metaphor.

Speaking of an unconscious mind and a conscious/aware mind implies a separation that does not in fact exist. These terms are chosen simply for linguistic convenience, since there is just one mind that governs the body. Your mind, an innate intelligence, connects intimately to your body. It organizes your inner life and controls automatic body functions. It serves you in planning and remembering and so on. You don't have to think about breathing, or secreting digestive enzymes, or producing immune system cells, although you can put your attention on these things and, for example, consciously choose to breathe slower or faster, like a Lamaze patient in the throes of labor. But much of the time, it's just as well to let the part of mind that operates the body run itself automatically.

The part of mind that thinks, reasons, and makes choices is where consciousness or awareness is most desirable. But, even here, your mind is not always conscious of its work. Your so-called conscious mind changes as you choose to pay attention. You engage in selective awareness. Just as a child engrossed in a TV show might not hear his mother calling him, you will not notice all the work—the thoughts and feelings—of your own mind. Similarly, your so-called unconscious mind expands or contracts as formerly unconscious processes surface and reach a level where you notice them, just as mom's yelling or turning the TV off causes the child to pay attention and get the message.

The unconscious mind is that part of your mind whose contents you are unaware of at any given time. Sometimes this is to your benefit: you don't have to think about all the millions of automatic processes needed to keep you functioning. You don't tell your digestive enzymes to flow or stop to think about breathing. Your internal operating system (akin to the disk operating system on a personal computer) handles this very well. Sometimes to your detriment unconscious material influences your choices and leads to negative behaviors. For example, if you are angry at your spouse and unable to admit your feelings, you might do something to undermine him—perhaps spill a glass of soda on him accidentally on purpose.

The human body is a network of billions of interconnected cells, each in communication with the others. You, as awareness, reside in that body. The body is the temple of the spirit, the house of the soul, and the reflection of the mind. Each cell, through a spark of consciousness, knows how to re-create itself. The intelligence within each cell is part of your so-called unconscious mind. If these cells receive a message about a headache, they can join together to create an ache in your head. In this sense, language becomes a connecting link among the cells in your body.

Psychologist Dr. Dennis Jaffe, writing in *Healing From Within* asks a key question, "Are specific diseases related to particular life crises, personality types or emotions?" He continues, "though I have studiously avoided proclaiming this connection as a reflection of reality, physicians have detected a link between emotions, personality, and specific illness for centuries. A growing number of recent studies have added support to this hypothesis."

Jaffe came to this conclusion after studying the work of psychosomatic experts W.J. Grace and D.T. Graham.[1] Jaffe wrote:

> Grace and Graham had conducted in-depth interviews with one hundred twenty-eight patients, each of whom had the symptoms of one of twelve different diseases. The researchers were trying to determine what life-situations were associated with attacks of the patients' symptoms. Certain emotional attitudes, they found, were related to the onset of symptoms of each specific disease. They speculated that, in effect, the patients were expressing physiologically what they felt was being done to them in their every day lives.

> For example, twenty-seven patients reported attacks of diarrhea when they wanted to end a particular situation, or to get rid of something or somebody. One man developed this symptom after purchasing a defective automobile, telling the researchers, 'If only I could get rid of it.' Defecation, of course, is ridding oneself of substances after the body is done with them.

> Another seventeen patients had constipation when they were grimly determined to persevere through a seemingly insurmountable problem. They used statements such as, 'This marriage is never going to be any better, but I won't quit.' And what is constipation but a bodily process of holding on to substances without change, despite discomfort?

Twelve patients with hay fever and seven with asthma articulated another set of attitudes. They faced a situation that they would rather not have had to confront, or that they wished would disappear. They wanted to hide from it, avoid it and divest themselves from all responsibility for it. Grace and Graham noted that these two syndromes—asthma and hay fever—often occurred together. They are both reactions to an external irritant in which the membranes of the nose and lungs swell up and narrow, in their attempt to dilute the irritant or wash it away. The body, just like the person, wants to get rid of something.

Thirty one patients suffered from urticaria, a skin reaction to trauma, leading to blistering and inflammation. The patients with this ailment felt they were being interfered with or prevented from doing something they wanted to do. And they could not find a way to deal effectively with their frustration. They were so preoccupied with the way that others interfered with them that it was as if they were being physically beaten by their adversaries—hence the skin blisters. This parallels the 'picked on' feeling of Ellerbroek's acne patients, who ironically, literally picked on themselves as well.

Nausea and vomiting (in eleven patients) occurred when a person wished something had never occurred. Ulcers (nine patients) were characterized by desires for revenge and getting even. Migraine headaches (fourteen patients) were provoked after a person had made an intense effort to complete a task. Hypertension was common among those who continually worried about meeting all possible threats (Type A behavior). Low back pain (eleven patients) was found among people who wanted to do something involving the whole body, usually running away."

This study dramatically supports the idea that your emotions can translate into body language, especially if you won't admit or act on your feelings. The feelings remain hidden, perhaps even from you, until they manifest in some illness.

Disease as Messenger

Physical sensations such as itching, crying, rashes, sweating, pain, pressure, orgasm, and smiles are all part of the language of the body. So is disease. During illness the body communicates whether our actions are detracting from or adding to our well-being.

Milton Ward, in a helpful book entitled *The Brilliant Function Of Pain,* wrote "Pain, rather than being a terror, is actually our own brilliant force, functioning in our behalf, ready to guide us through life if we are but willing to listen."[22] Pain transmits a powerful message from body to mind. In this way it serves to communicate the way to health. Disease is your body's way of talking to you, telling you that something isn't working, showing you graphically and sometimes painfully that something is amiss.

When you are "diseasing," your body is actually attempting to heal itself by correcting imbalances and restoring harmony. Feeling bad is often the route to getting better. During acne-ing, for example, the skin pushes out toxins that aren't removed through the primary channels of elimination. A cold eliminates excess mucus, an effect of poor eating, environmental pressures, and other stresses and strains on the body. Even the rash of chicken pox contains toxic, contagious material that the body is eliminating. A tumor is your body's attempt to encapsulate cells grown awry. Perhaps your body doesn't have the strength to eliminate this threat any other way.

Spiritual Growth through Illness

Life-threatening and chronic degenerative illnesses can result from negative thoughts and feelings, among other known causes. Disease, rather than an event to be feared, is frequently a positive force enabling us to see what changes are necessary to improve ourselves. We make the necessary changes by taking charge of our behaviors. We take charge when we realize that we act out through disease our conscious and unconscious beliefs and thought patterns. When we look at our illness and other crises in the context of this larger picture we can grow spiritually and emotionally.

Erik Esselstyn, Ed.D., then a counselor at the world-famous Gesell Institute of Human Development in New Haven, was a guest speaker during one of my courses. During a bout with cancer, he faced his emotions and changed his thinking. Erik was then dean of students at a college in North Carolina. The experience changed his career path. He and his wife Micki now offer seminars and workshops on wellness, releasing anger, and creating life changes because of major illness. Micki says, "We have cancer to thank for a lot—it made us appreciate life." Erik teaches, "A key element in achieving and maintaining good health is the acceptance of personal responsibility for our own actions, gracefully acknowledging the fact that *each one of us is responsible for putting on his own seat belt."*

Accepting Responsibility

Many people aren't aware of their power to make themselves sick or to heal themselves. Your initial response to the idea that you cause your own disease might be skepticism, fear, anger, or dismay. Skepticism is reasonable. If your reaction is fear, anger, or dismay, it might be worthwhile to examine the source of your feelings. Perhaps you feel that way because you equate responsibility with blame and shame. You may not be used to forgiving yourself for your mistakes, changing to more appropriate behavior, and then forgetting about it. Some people think they have to act perfectly and when they don't, they punish and berate themselves with negative self-talk and feelings of guilt.

We are not victims. Rather, when we forget to take responsibility for our health, we often choose unconsciously to harm ourselves. Then we feel like victims of the fates. There is a better way of thinking available. But, it takes awareness and practice. You don't have to roll over and play dead. When you choose to be responsible for your own health and well-being, there is a lot you can do to help yourself. The aware use of the guiding light in your mind is a powerful way to help yourself to be well.

Self-Help Experience #7
Giving Reasons

Purpose: To uncover your beliefs related to any illness, problem, or conflict in your life. These questions will begin to illuminate some of the underlying factors behind symptoms.

Ask yourself or have someone else ask you:

1.   What might have caused your current problem?

2.   What threat and/or loss does it represent to you?

3. What is the payoff (if any) or gain you get from having this problem?

4. How do you believe the problem should be treated? Include any medical or non-medical treatments you think would help you.

5. Have you ever been ill before at this same time of year?

6. Did your problem begin around the anniversary of some traumatic event like a death, divorce, car accident, hospitalization, etc.? This could even refer to an event many years past.

7. Do you want to rid yourself of this problem? Why?

8. Do you want to change yourself or someone else? Why?

9. What is this illness trying to teach you? Can you live with and learn from this problem? What could you learn?

10. Are you willing to resolve this conflict? If yes, What would it take? If no, Why not?

Self-Help Experience #8
21 Questions to Inventory Your Feelings

Purpose: To take an inventory of your common beliefs and attitudes about a variety of everyday experiences and events in order to uncover your feelings about them[23]

Many people go through life denying—not feeling—their feelings. Since disease often results from ignored feelings acting on the body like underground invaders, it is important to allow these feelings to surface. Pay attention to your feelings as you read each question. Your "gut reactions" will be evidence of underground feelings that might affect you. It is possible to change the way you experience your body and the way your body reacts to you.

Ask yourself:

1. What do you expect from people?

2. Do you have a high or low opinion of most people?

3. Do most people take advantage of you or are they usually fair with you?

5. Are most people honest or dishonest?

6. How do you value your relationships?

7. Is work generally satisfying or frustrating?

8. How do you value your work?

9. Are you generally optimistic or pessimistic?

10. Do you expect life to serve you or do you in?

11. Do you feel you give more to others, or receive more from others?

13. Do you have enough money to satisfy your basic needs? Your desires?

14. Would more money make you happier?

15. Do you give generously?

16. Do you have integrity? Do you keep your word?

17. Do you generally like yourself?

18. Do you often feel "guilty"?

19. Is life often "too much to bear"?

20. Do you frequently desire revenge?

21. Do you often think... "What if?" "Why me?" "If only"?

Self-Help Experience #9
Choosing Thoughts: The Worry Wart Exercise

Purpose: To practice being in charge of what you think about

Instructions

1. *Choose* to think some upsetting thoughts. *Worry* about something or someone. Think about something that makes you feel angry.

2. Stop thinking these thoughts. Tell yourself: "I release these upsetting thoughts and choose to think some happy thoughts." For example: Recall a happy incident. Think about someone you love. Imagine yourself winning a lot of money, or achieving a long-desired goal. Remember that God loves you.

3. Notice the difference in the way you *feel* when you are thinking these different types of thoughts.

4. Tell yourself, "I have the power to choose what I will think about." Do this whenever you find yourself beset by worries or negative thoughts.

I should have my head examined
Get your hopes up.
Stick your neck out

Core Beliefs
and Seedthoughts

4

Recent research has shown that much illness is self-created. Words are often the trigger (catalyst) that lead to the symptoms of disease: you are what you think, feel, and say about yourself. You are what you believe about you. Language is a visible link between the physical reality of the body and the emotional reality and thoughts of the mind.

Emotions have both physical and mental expressions. The language of the mind is expressed in words and pictures through talking, writing, dreaming, mental imagining, visualizing, and fantasizing. The language of the body is expressed through both unpleasant and pleasant physical sensations like itching, sweating, rashes, pain, pressure, tears, laughter, smiles, orgasms, energy, and exuberance. Even a sneeze is part of the language connection, a loud clearly expressed response arising from a bodily need. Gross reactions to strong emotions include cold feet, sweaty palms, and the flush of excitement, among others.

A *"seedthought"* is a significant catalyst for a physical or emotional response. A seedthought is a thought you think frequently that either emanates from, or creates, your core beliefs. Just as the apple core contains seeds that sprout into an apple tree, you have, at your core, beliefs which shape you.

Core beliefs are the basic assumptions and ideas upon which your everyday thoughts and actions are based. These deeply held values lead to almost reflex-like knee jerk actions in response to circumstances and events in your life. You may not be conscious of your core beliefs and their accompanying seedthoughts; but your core belief system affects every part of your being—physical, mental, emotional, and spiritual. *Core beliefs can be altered by using consciously chosen seedthoughts.*

Seedthoughts include the attitudes and emotions surrounding the thought. These seem to determine the potency of the seedthought, just as the soil around the seed determines the strength and vitality of the plant. A seedthought is an idea planted through the mind that grows into manifestation in the body. A seedthought can be health-promoting or, like a weed, choke out the life around it. The body expresses in physical form both the positive and negative output of the mind. Thoughts and emotions stick to it, just as bits of salt stick to a pretzel, adding flavor and seasoning. Some seasoning enhances our experience of the pretzel. But too much salt often spoils the taste. So too, too much of certain types of thoughts and emotions can negatively affect the body.

Flakes as Feedback

Before I started to write this book, I was plagued by a persistent case of dandruff. Months of aggressive treatment failed to eliminate the ugly white flakes. Then I decided to see if there was a language connection. I soon had the answer.

For years, I had been involved in the presentation of new ideas such as women's liberation, holistic health, and spiritual healing. Frequently, while presenting these ideas, I would think: "They think I'm flaky." When I realized how clearly that thought was affecting me, I gasped. "They think I'm flaky" was a thought that seemed to be the source of my dandruff. It seemed a perfect example of the creative role of language in the reactions and behaviors of my body. When I recognized the creative power of words I first coined the term "seedthought."

What I had to do next was to verify that eliminating the seedthought would eliminate the physical condition connected to it. Recognizing the untruthfulness of "They think I'm flaky," I canceled the thought whenever it occurred to me. I realized that whether or not others saw me that way, the thought "I'm flaky" *originated in my own mind and was solely my responsibility.* Then I projected it onto others, creating a stubborn case of dandruff flakes in the process. I told myself the real truth, "I am not flaky! I am serious, thoughtful, fun, loving, and committed to new ideas. Many people who interact with me know that." Within two weeks of my initial recognition of the flaky seedthought, and without further treatment, the dandruff disappeared. I had altered the belief underlying my seedthought when I acknowledged to myself that people did take me seriously. When I knew I wasn't flaky, I stopped flaking.

Since each person is unique, you might have different dandruff-related core beliefs; if you have dandruff, you might have a quite different seedthought. It is also possible to heal your unwanted condition without discovering a specific seedthought. Healing is self-induced when you recognize your responsibility and take appropriate physical, mental, and spiritual action.

Our Internal Chatter

The *Body* is a remarkable vehicle which allows us to feel physical sensations of pleasure and pain so we can learn from our experience.

The *Mind* speaks to us with words, pictures, or images (seedthoughts) which can translate into physical conditions in the body.

The *Spirit* is the life force within a body—the breath of life. We learn spiritual lessons related to love, compassion, and trust using mind and body. We are taught by feeling bodily experiences. Mind helps us to understand and create meaning, enabling us to grow as human (physical) and spiritual beings. *Spirit is the part of us that observes, knows, grows, and loves.*

By observing our bodily reactions, we can discover seedthoughts and core beliefs which lurk beneath our conscious awareness. Seedthoughts like "I am flaky" are potent triggers that stimulate physical and emotional reactions in the body.

John Graham is a former NATO negotiator who now heads The Giraffe Project, an organization that acknowledges pioneers who "stick their necks out" by taking risks to improve the world. He told me, "I healed a persistent ache in my left foot by moving professionally in the right direction." Just as the oyster turns the irritating grain of sand into a pearl, so too, humans can turn irritating experiences into experiences of personal growth.

Decoding Sensations

An intelligent approach to symptoms is to try and decode the meaning of the sensations in order to understand how to help your body. First check the physical basis of a sensation: Is it organic or is it functional? *Organic* means the sensation arises from the living tissue of the body. There is verifiable change or damage to a specific body part.

Functional pertains to dis-ease having no apparent physiological or structural cause. Something isn't working right and there is no known reason why. An example of this is *idiopathic* (unknown cause) *hypertension* (high blood pressure). For hypertension there are several tests—for example, kidney X rays— a doctor would use to try and determine the reason for the elevated blood pressure. If no physical cause is found, the disease is considered idiopathic. Helpful medical advice would then include a lifestyle re-assessment with suggestions for dietary changes, exercise, and tension-reducing activities. Exploring emotions is a useful part of this process. In any idiopathic disease, an exploration of the mental and emotional language connections can yield significant insights.

When I first wrote the above paragraph I began looking for my own hypertension-related seedthoughts. I felt *pressured* to find some. "Grin and bear it," "Keep a stiff upper lip," and "Grit your teeth" are some I've come up with so far. And I'm still looking.

If you have a pain in the ribcage area, it might be caused by a cracked rib—an organic condition. If you've eliminated that possibility, emotion or negative attitudes might be causing discomfort there. Your body usually reflects your underlying emotional condition. Tightness in the gut might relate to emotional tenseness as well as to problems from food, viruses, or other physical causes. Physical indigestion often results from the stress of emotional indigestion.

When decoding the meaning behind a symptom, *first rule out physical causes* and then look for emotional causes. Explore the emotional reasons for your dis-ease by searching for seedthoughts. If you often suffer from physical indigestion, examine your emotions to see if there is something in your life that "eats away at you" or "lies heavy in your gut." Perhaps you haven't "digested the meaning of an experience" or "assimilated an important life lesson." Maybe you are upset and "eating your heart out." Use your body's speech as a guide to the unconscious part of your mind. Then act on what you've discovered.

Several years ago I had a severe rash. The itching and burning related to my anger, frustration, and impatience to get on with more important work—this book, for instance. But since there were other things I needed to do first, I had to learn patience. Recognizing the connection between my emotions and the allergic reactions helped me to accept and release the underlying frustration, which helped my healing. Eventually I saw that I was actually working on the book all along. My ailments were part of the research process.

By witnessing sensations and symptoms in your body, your underlying pattern of beliefs becomes clear. Objective witnessing requires practice. It means observing, decoding, and understanding without negative self-judgment, blame, or punishment. If you are sick, you need to:

Learn from the experience.
Forgive yourself.
And move on.

Through the sensations in my body I often discover painful emotions. If I direct my energy and attention to a particular area, it usually begins to improve. Sometimes the problem first intensifies, just as using soap and water to clean a dirty shirt at first increases the mess, till dirt and soap wash out together.

Some days a pain in my gut reflects the hurt and unhappiness I feel or perhaps try to avoid feeling. Then I am literally *feeling* my feelings. Noticing my thoughts verifies the honesty of my body, as I discover what I am really thinking and feeling about something or someone.

Other days I almost purr like a kitten, reflecting a more positive state of mind. Since knowing myself and becoming a better person is my goal, I am grateful for the learning my body provides. An attitude of gratitude is important in the process of self-healing.

Chronic recurrences of a particular symptom may well be the result of a well-defined mental blueprint. Different parts of the body speak to, as well as for, different people. Although there are typical patterns that many people exhibit, we each will have our own unique reactive language. For some who feel burdened, for instance, the back might act up. They have "too much to shoulder" or are "weighted down" with responsibility. For others, these same feelings might manifest as trouble with the weight-bearing parts—the joints of the leg, the knee, foot, or ankle.

Cliches as Emotional Expressions

Cliches often become seedthoughts. These seedthoughts express emotion using words whose meaning relates directly to the symptoms evoked. For example, an expression most of us have used at one time or another is, "That____is a real pain in the neck, head, gut, or ass" (you fill in the blank). We are generally expressing our feelings about some particular thing or situation. But saying "that is a real pain in the whatever" can actually trigger a painful stiff neck, an upset stomach, or a headache. Your spoken words may match a particular symptom exactly, triggering that symptom as a sensation (dis-ease) in your body.

The process also works in reverse. You may begin using those expressions after you first physically feel something amiss. For example, if you have real physical distress from a stiff neck or an upset stomach, you may want to talk about how you feel. So saying "that was a pain in the neck" or "that gave me an upset stomach" is true; you do already have a sore neck or an upset stomach. The seedthought stimulating your physical distress *is then reinforced by the distress* as you feel it, strengthening your original symptom-triggering thought. Your *belief* in whatever that _____ is that gives you such distress is stored in your unconscious mind. Then just thinking the seedthought "that _____ will give me whatever" can trigger the physical distress. But discovery of the seedthought can break the sickness cycle.

"My nerves are raw" is another statement many people use to express some kind of upset. But that seedthought too can be stored in the mind, and later "solidified" in the body, resulting in pain and inflammation. Here too, the words used match the actual symptoms present in many diseases, among them the painful condition called arthritis. The nerves can be raw and painful in the body of an arthritis sufferer. Your body often takes your words quite literally and creates what you've spoken of.

In order to move from being a victim to a victor, it is necessary to mentally recognize and accept your feelings and then eliminate any negative verbal expressions. Like Charlie Brown, don't keep asking, "Why's everybody always pickin' on me?"

A common seedthought for some people is a name. The mere mention of someone we love deeply can bring feelings of joy, love, pleasure, or fear of loss. The loss of a loved one can result in pain and despair when remembering the beloved. Even if the relationship ended because you wanted to end it, the name can retain the power to evoke a physical or emotional reaction.

Any thought can stimulate us. However, we each have basic seedthoughts which stimulate predictable reactions whenever we think that thought. An example of this occurs in people prone to the panic of acute anxiety. Just thinking they are on the verge of anxiety can lead them to the sensations of anxiety. The body has learned that sweating, shaking, tight muscles, and nausea are some of the sensations that accompany anxiety and it will produce those symptoms in the presence of the seedthought "I am having an anxiety attack."

Neurology and psychiatry professor Viktor Frankl calls this "anticipatory anxiety."[24] An individual afraid of stuttering when speaking is more likely to stutter. Frankl wrote of the irony that *fear makes come true what one is afraid of and what one forcibly wishes for often brings the opposite result.* "The more a man tries to demonstrate his sexual potency or a woman her ability to experience orgasm, the less they are able to succeed." A fearful expectation often leads right to the undesirable result; wanting something so much, yet believing it won't happen, can block its happening.

Which Comes First, Chicken or Egg?

Notice how you explain your physical sensations. You may tell yourself you are sick or you may tell yourself you are well. Sometimes you ignore physical sensations, but *subconsciously, every thought tells your body how to react.* Each thought promotes health or illness. The internal dialogue goes on in drumbeat time whether you hear it or not. Once an idea has gained a foothold in your physical world, other thoughts, words and images may affect its existence.

Words are not the sole cause of dis-ease. But, they certainly are a link in a chain of causative factors that also includes environment, lifestyle, and heredity. Words create the climate that allows disease to flourish. Language affects the quality of life.

There is no final, definitive evidence yet that the words you speak actually cause disease or whether they simply reflect what is already present. There appears to be some truth in both these points of view. *At times, we develop physical disease just to allow us to experience our thoughts and emotions, so that we can recognize and change them.* Thus, your language connection works two ways:

Sometimes your emotions become physical problems;
Sometimes your physical problems lead you to recognize your emotions.

We don't always know which comes first, the chicken or the egg, the thought or the emotion, the disease or the feelings. And people do recognize their language connection whenever they use that common old saying, "I should have my head examined."

Self-Help Experience #10
Self-Awareness

Purpose: To expand your ability to recognize your seedthoughts and core beliefs; to learn how your memories affect you; to recognize thoughts on which you may have patterned your life

Instructions

1. Have a paper and pen handy so that you can write down your discoveries at the end of this exercise. Once you are comfortably settled, after having read through all the instructions, close your eyes for a few moments to block out any external stimuli. This exercise works with eyes opened or closed. But, if you have trouble recognizing your feelings, then closing your eyes will improve your results.

2. *Notice how you are feeling right now.* Observe your thoughts, feelings and any physical sensations. Describe to yourself the way different parts of your body feel. Do you have uncomfortable physical sensations? What is your emotional state? Are you happy, sad, angry, bored, excited, curious, interested, or something else? As you follow the rest of these instructions, notice any changes.

3. *Think about some thing, incident, or person that made you angry.* Become aware of all the details of the scene: who was there, what they were wearing, the colors around you, where you were, the expressions on people's faces, and so on. Really remember what anger was like and describe your physical sensations as you think about your anger. Notice if you can re-experience the anger in your mind, to see how it feels physically and emotionally.

    See if your sensations change as you allow yourself to remember and observe your experience. Sometimes an emotion like anger will disappear after a few moments and be replaced by another emotion, perhaps sadness, or even compassion.

4. *Recall a time when you were happy.* Recall in detail what went on at that time. Really remember what happy was like and describe your physical sensations as you think about being happy. Notice if you can re-experience that time in your mind, to see how it feels physically and emotionally.

5. *Think of the name of someone you love.* How do that name and the image of that person make you feel? Describe your physical sensations as you think about your loved one.

6. *Now remember someone you once loved, but who is no longer in your life.* See how that makes you feel. Describe your physical sensations as you think about this person.

Observe your physical sensations, thoughts, and feelings as you examine any situation in your life that upsets you. Use this process to release emotion whenever you need to be clear-headed. Do this when you are problem solving or prior to major lifestyle changes such as a new job, a new home, marriage or divorce, and so on.

When you become aware of how your memories and underlying beliefs are affecting you right now, you will be motivated to make the changes that will improve your life. The rest of this book and many of the exercises to come will help you to make those changes that mend the mind and heal the body. There are many techniques for you to use to help you to "think yourself healthy." But, becoming aware by observing yourself living your life is effective even by itself.

Self-Help Experience #11
Changing Upsetting Thoughts

Purpose: To give you practice in changing your mind to control the effects of or to harmonize your emotions. Being upset will simply add more power and energy to a negative thought, thus reinforcing it. You can abort an anxiety attack with this technique.

Instructions

1. *Release a negative thought by saying a particular word or phrase, like "cancel," "God forbid," or "delete."* You are simply giving your brain, the computer, a command to abort whatever is going on right now. Your internal dialogue might go: "This project is a headache. Cancel, cancel."

    After you cancel, replace the negative thought with a positive one of your choosing. For example: "This project is very challenging." From this perspective, you will be reprogramming your mind in a more positive way.

2. *Visualize (imagine) yourself taking an eraser and erasing the thought.* Then consciously create a positive image to replace the erased thought. For example, first visualize your previous negative image of a specific project. In your mind's eye, see the image being rubbed away by your mental eraser. In the place of the previous image, picture an image of what the successfully completed project would look like. You might then see yourself celebrating the successful completion of your challenging project.

I sometimes had trouble writing when my mind created thoughts of failure, leading me to fear and frustration. After noting those feelings, I'd release the stimulus thoughts and change my mind. I spent many happy moments imagining this manuscript done, finding an agent, and finally being published.

I *saw* the completed book. I *felt* my happiness. I imagined myself on TV and signing autographs in bookstores. Pretending like this often motivated me to write when I felt like doing something else.

That breaks my heart
I'm itching to get on with it
My head isn't screwed on straight

Emotion and
Your Body's Language

5

I discovered the true power of seedthoughts by observing and experiencing my body and then noticing what I was thinking and saying. For example, I used to say, "I don't have my head on straight," referring to my emotional life. I paid no attention then to the literal meaning of my words. I used those words as a feeble excuse for some imperfection in my behavior. I thought this was a good idea, but this belittling myself, putting myself down, was really a self-defeating habit.

Then, one day in 1976, I tripped while walking in the woods. My neck and the muscles holding my spine in place felt sore. Being cautious, I went to a chiropractor for treatment. I thought I would be fine. But a week later, while walking in New York City, I felt something in my neck move, heard a crunching noise, and experienced intense fear.

Over the next few days I noticed my neck sloping off at an angle. To counterbalance the angle of my neck, the weight of my head went towards the opposite direction. "My head is not on straight" had become an accurate statement about my body. I became aware of the language connection between my body and my crooked neck when I finally noticed how frequently I talked about not being straight. I don't talk that way anymore. Which came first, the injury or the statement? I honestly don't remember.

Dr. Robert Marshall, a chiropractor, provides a similar example of how beliefs can affect the body:

> A new patient came to me for an adjustment. Her body was very misaligned. One shoulder was considerably higher than the other. She looked almost crooked. I suggested that she go home and look at herself in the mirror.
>
> When she returned for her next visit, she shared her astonishment at really looking at her body and seeing for the first time how crookedly she presented herself to the world. Looking in the mirror she discovered a seedthought taught to her in childhood: 'Don't be straight with people.' She saw those words clearly reflected in her crooked body. This patient told me that she had considerable difficulty in being with people. She never was straight with them, even though she wanted to be. Her family taught her dishonesty by telling her not to be up front with people. 'Keep your feelings to yourself. Don't show your hand. Never be straight with people.' Consequently, facing people straight and looking them in the eye was difficult. And her body was very crooked.

Emotional Connections to the Past

During my childhood my mother repeated over and over, "If you don't have something nice to say, don't say it." As a result, I was prone to hide certain "not nice" feelings from others, turning them inward upon myself. I too was taught not to be straight with people, and I too have a body that isn't straight. Hiding feelings and storing them in my body required a great deal of energy, resulting in excess stress and muscle tension. Resentment builds up quickly. Sometimes I'd explode and dump on those I love.

Now I am learning to release these feelings by being more straight with people from the beginning. Being straight with people appears to be a major issue in my life. I don't mean to criticize my mother for teaching me to speak kindly. But, I really don't have to hide my feelings. I can express them in a way that is helpful to others. Expressing anger or disappointment can be useful feedback to the recipient, especially if tempered with love.

Writer Tony Schwartz describes the following experience: "Three years ago, I was suffering from chronic back pain despite two years of visits to every imaginable kind of specialist. Finally I went to see a doctor named John Sarno, at NYU's Rusk Institute, who believes that virtually all back pain is due not to structural causes but to stress. Sarno treats back pain by giving a series of lectures on the physiology and psychology of tension. He teaches the power of the mind over the body. Period. My pain went away within several weeks and has never returned. I have since sent more than forty back-pain sufferers to Sarno, including at least a half-dozen with herniated disks. All but one of the forty were pain-free within a matter of weeks."[25]

Memories also trigger bodily sensations. Memory, in fact, is attached to emotion. We tend to remember those experiences that initially elicited a strong emotional reaction in us. Names of people important to us from the past and in the present can become seedthoughts. The name can evoke a physical response and emotional reaction because it symbolizes feelings related to love or loss of love.

I recently saw a man with whom I had shared a very emotional year. I was excited and nervous about seeing him again. Our friendship was deep, perhaps more so because we weren't lovers. Although I was relieved when the relationship ended, the pain at the end was strong. The mere thought of him or hearing his name triggered a physical reaction in me. I'd feel like I was being punched from within, with a tightness in my gut, pressure and heat in my chest, and a heart that would start racing. His name and my image of him had become a seedthought.

For a whole year after we stopped meeting, I processed and released my emotions associated with that relationship. I was very unhappy, mourning the pain of other lost loves as I experienced long-suppressed emotions. It is common for unexpressed grief to be stored in the body and triggered by fresh loss. The release of grief was definitely health-producing.

I thought I was completely healed of the hurt and no longer missed him, but I was uncertain of my subconscious reaction to being with him. After seeing him I felt fine, but still I wondered if I was fooling myself, suppressing my emotions, still missing him. A dream symbolically showed me I was really okay. In my dream we sat in a car, preparing to go to a movie. We acknowledged our love for each other. Then I kissed him goodbye, saying, "I choose to be somewhere else—not with you." Then I left the car. This dream confirmed that I am okay whether I see him or not.

The effect of grief on the body is reported in the medical literature. James Lynch, a doctor specializing in psychosomatic medicine, makes a strong case for the effects of grief and separation on the human heart. He notes that "Drs. Kraus and Lillienfeld, in 1959, using data published by the National Office of Vital Statistics, were among the first to call attention to the abrupt rise in mortality among widows and widowers, especially in the young widowed group."[26] People do express their grief in their bodies and they can and do die of "broken hearts."

Researchers Kiecolt and Glaser reported on a variety of studies of immunological changes related to divorce and separation. In one study, they found that those women who had been separated one year or less had poorer immune function than a well-matched control group of married women. It was also reported that people with fewer close relationships have higher rates of disease and death.[27] What happens in one's interpersonal relationships does have health consequences.

You Are the Meaning Maker

Emotions and your overall sense of illness or well-being are felt and expressed in your body. Your general feeling of illness or wellness is a purely subjective evaluation which you make for yourself. Often it relates to your general emotional state. You can physically feel, as well as speak of or act out, the emotions of happiness, joy, anger, sadness, or grief. You feel happiness when you laugh or smile. Anger is felt as muscle tension, a churning in the gut, or even a rise in body temperature. Tears give physical expression to sadness, joy, or grief.

You, as the maker of meaning, can discover the *why* of each physical sensation. Pay attention to your body and think about what a feeling means. Body conditions reflect emotional attitudes. So, people with severe illness such as heart disease, cancer, arthritis, or even AIDS, should be treated for underlying emotional distress.

Even if their seedthoughts remain a mystery, healing will still be facilitated.

Seedthoughts often interconnect, forming a pattern for the body. More than one set of thoughts may be responsible for triggering the form, shape, and condition of your body. Similarly, a series of interconnected beliefs can affect your emotions. Eliminating any one seedthought can have the effect of toppling the whole dis-easing structure. But more extensive work might be necessary in order to change the negative blueprint which you have been using to create your physical and emotional reality.

Citing innumerable studies and case histories, Paul Pearsall demonstrates the roles of mind and emotion in all disease, the crucial link between your state of mind and your health, and the need to allow healing to occur by knowing, loving, and accepting yourself. He writes, "Epidemiology, the study of large numbers of people and emerging patterns of disease, also points to the importance of the psychosomatic relationship. In 1976, Dr. C.B. Thomas published results of a study of medical students who were followed for thirty years. She found that profiles of psychological tests were predictive of such sicknesses as cancer, heart disease and high blood pressure. Dr. George Valiant conducted a similar study published in 1974 and 1977. In his study, a large population of Harvard students was followed for thirty years, and the relationship between emotional maturity and disease vulnerability was clearly shown."[28]

There is scientific evidence of a direct physical mechanism uniting the brain, the mind, the emotions and the immune system. Messenger molecules called neuropeptides, transmitted through virtually all the body fluids (blood, lymph, etc.) seem to link the immune, endocrine, and central nervous systems.

Networks of Seedthoughts

Examining my physical sensations, I often recognize emotions I was unconscious of feeling. Frequently, I discover many seedthoughts that are interconnected—my own negative blueprint. Several language connections became apparent to me at a time when I was being "attacked" by body rashes. Three times in six weeks, I broke out in a horrendous rash all over my body. I itched.

I burned. There is still some scarring on my back from that time. The rashes seemed to result from food allergies. But equally, the rashes were messages resulting from deeply felt, but unrecognized emotions.

My doctor reassured me that the condition was not a serious disease. It looked and felt worse than it actually was. After a while I was able to see the experience as an opportunity to learn about myself and transform my relationship to the part of me that is my body. *Being itchy* related to being impatient. *Burning up* expressed my unacknowledged anger in a physical way. I felt ugly and unclean.

"Hexaba" is a name I use to refer to the ugly, bad part of me—the seething network of unexpressed negative emotions and seedthoughts. She was in my unconscious, screaming to get out, to be accepted and loved. She expressed herself through my body and conceptualizing her was my attempt to make a painful life-experience meaningful.

I kept saying how ugly the rash was, but I didn't hide. Wearing makeup was out of the question. My skin was too sensitive, my lips cracked and burned. I often asked my family to look at the rash: "How does it look? Is it improving or getting worse?" There was a dichotomy between believing I looked ugly and wanting everyone to see me. I attended a wedding and had my picture taken in order to remember that time. Soon the ugliness I felt inside was leaving. My skin was a mirror of what was going on inside me. I was learning, through the reflection provided by my skin and the loving concern of friends and family, to love, accept, and forgive myself. It wasn't the first, nor the last, time that my body was my teacher.

I recognized that I was responsible for this rash, perhaps because of erratic and overindulgent food habits, as well as embedded patterns of self-hate. Discovering the food connection helped me heal the rash and the physical behaviors stemming from my underlying emotional pattern. My body's suffering made me more aware of certain problem areas and provided me with an incentive for deeper self-examination, change, and transformation.

As I recognized my seedthoughts, I created mental antidotes to change my unhealthy core beliefs and alter my emotional reactions. I would frequently repeat positive affirmations to myself in order to counteract the harmful core beliefs. I also played video games in my mind, visualizing "Pacmen" coursing through my body; clearing out foreign invaders; gobbling up germs, allergens, tumors, and fats. Soon afterward, the rashes on my body disappeared and I lost fifteen pounds. These mental processes were used in conjunction with physical techniques such as an altered diet, exercising, and herbal remedies. The seedthoughts and core beliefs I discovered—and their antidotes—included:

Seedthought and Symptom: I am itching.
Core Belief: I felt emotionally at odds with myself. I was itching to move on to the next cycle in my life, to begin writing this book.
Mental Antidote: I am moving as fast as I really want to. I am more patient each day.

Seedthought and Symptom: I am burning up. The rash was so red hot it burned my skin.
Core Belief: Burning up was indicative to me of my stored anger burning me as it was released through my skin.
Mental Antidote: I transform the warmth within to love and peace. I am cool and at ease.

Seedthought and Symptom: I am ugly. The rash was gross looking.
Core Belief: I felt as if poison was coming out of me both physically and spiritually; the poison of self-hate and anger.
Mental Antidote: I am beautiful and purifying my soul.

During my rash experience I checked with an internist and a dermatologist to rule out serious organic disease. There was no specific medical treatment but the dermatologist reassured me that this condition wasn't as serious as it appeared, just ugly and uncomfortable. He said, "This too shall pass," a reassuring affirmation. Who is to say which of the things I did was most responsible for my healing? The one thing I am sure of was that I learned a lot about myself and grew emotionally from this experience.

The skin is an easily viewed mirror of our unconscious state. It can be restored to health by changing our thinking. Pearsall writes of a boy with a so-called incurable skin condition called congenital ichthyosiform erythrodermia, which results in hardening and blackening of the skin. He writes, "All major dermatology textbooks report no known cure for this terrible disease. Hypnotist Dr. Mason saw the boy and offered mental imagery suggestions to relax him and to help him learn to see his skin as becoming normal. Within ten days the skin had returned to normal. Dr. Mason's results, published in the *British Medical Journal,* were later verified by three other medical researchers." Other physicians later obtained positive results in improving other skin disorders. Concludes Pearsall, "We now know that 'T-cell-mediated skin response' relates to our emotions and beliefs, that the skin reacts intensely to our feelings."[29]

Jack, a former student of mine, often talked angrily as if he was "itching to clobber someone." All the while he was scratching the white scaly patches on his arms. In many ways a gentle soul who would never knowingly hurt anyone, Jack's anger was nevertheless intense. Unwilling to face himself as the true source of this anger, Jack's skin provided an outlet for his emotions. With no place to go, it "oozed out of his body," leading to the ugly, itchy rash of psoriasis.

Mind Over Matter

Dr. Barbara Brown used her background in brain and behavior research in her book *Supermind: The Ultimate Energy.* But her personal experience was useful too. After being told that she required a tonsillectomy, she spent time preparing her emotions before surgery. She wrote: "From time to time I would silently tell myself that the operation would be easy, cause no pain, and that there would be no problems." The operation, done without anesthetic, went well, she "felt no pain, didn't bleed and had absolutely no recovery problems. Mind over matter. This hidden capacity of mind to control the vital functions of the body has been useful to me at other times, although I confess I do not know what happens in the mind to accomplish such remarkable effects. I do know that I *will* it...."

Another time Brown nearly amputated her thumb in a household accident. After a surgeon sewed up the damage, she returned home, without stopping for pain pills. Again using the power of her mind, she repeatedly told herself that she would feel no pain. Because the surgeon had warned her that the thumb would be numb and disfigured, she added the command for the thumb to heal whole again, without scars. Between her mental suggestions and a few stiff drinks, she kept the pain at bay. "The thumb healed quickly, with only a faint line as reminder."[30]

These past ten years I have come to know myself better by observing my thoughts, experiencing my feelings, and seeing the effect of each on my body. This self-awareness enables me to live a happier, more peaceful, productive life. It has also become abundantly clear that *words are mental things which we embody with meaning.* We can unmask our body and discover the meaning it has. Just as we can *uncover* seedthoughts to find the patterns leading to disease in our body, we can *choose* seedthoughts to create newer, healthier patterns to live by. *If our words and thoughts can make us ill, they can also make us well.*

Self-Help Experience #12
Mirror Feedback

Purpose: To gather information about you by really looking at your body; to provide practice in observing yourself and seeing yourself as you look to others. This experience is strictly to gather information. This enhanced self-awareness often leads to healing without doing anything.

Instructions

1. *Stand naked in front of a full length mirror.* Take several deep breaths to relax your body. Observe the way your body looks, without trying to make it look better. Is it straight? Is one shoulder higher than the other? Do you slouch?

   The mirror facilitates self-observance because some people never look at themselves as they really are. They will suck in their tummy, or stand tall or smile to make themselves look better.

2. *Notice any thoughts you have while you are looking at your body.* If you are judging your body, notice how the judgments make you feel. When you have finished observing yourself, thank your body for supporting you throughout your life.

Self-Help Experience #13
Names as Seedthoughts

Purpose: To realize the power of memories

Instructions

1. Close your eyes. Relax. Repeat the name of someone who has been very important in your life. The image of that person, or the thought of that name, probably evokes powerful emotions within—perhaps joy, or sadness, or even anger. Your body is smart; it knows the physical sensations to produce.

2. Use your own name as a positive seedthought. Look in the mirror and tell yourself, "I love and appreciate you (say your name). Add a reason. For example, I might say, "I love and appreciate you, Barbara, because you are willing to dredge up your unconscious emotions and write about them to help others." The more reasons you can come up with the better. Do this as a daily exercise when you brush your teeth.

Something is eating away at me
Eat your heart out
It's a bitter pill to swallow

The Body as Emotional Barometer

6

At one time I believed I had a "stomach like a rock," that I could digest anything without stomach upset. The positive side of the seedthought "I have a stomach like a rock" comes from the notion that a strong stomach can "take it," implying also a strong person who can "take it." This belief reflected what I thought was my healthy digestive system. Then, at age 34, gallstones were found. The accepted treatment at the time was the removal of the gallbladder and I duly underwent that operation.

I then began to notice food-related problems and paid more attention to what I ate. Years later, during a meditation I recognized the language connection between the seedthought "stomach like a rock" and my digestive difficulties. Rocks are actually heavy and indigestible. Carrying rocks around is a burden. Early on, the seedthought helped me to believe I was invulnerable to poor eating. But actually, I needed to be careful about the food I ingested physically and the thoughts I ingested emotionally. When I ate foolishly and had fearful thoughts, I developed digestive problems. When I released negativity and worry, my digestive difficulties eased. This release is vital. One Eastern mystic dramatized it with the words, "If you are happy enough, you can digest rocks." My body has been an excellent vehicle for learning about the language connection.

Eating Right to Stay Fit

My involvement in holistic healing led me to work on improving my body through better nutrition. For years I followed a vegetarian health food diet, not worrying much about my digestion. By studying with different teachers, I learned many alternative approaches to eating. Among the eating plans I tried were the Grafs' low stress system, Macrobiotics, Natural Hygiene, the Pritikin diet, and a raw food and vegetable juice diet. Some things were common to all—mostly vegetarian and no sugar—but there were major differences. I was often very confused about what to eat.

In my quest for better health, I tried each new eating plan believing it would improve my health. I knew people who successfully used each one. My ever-improving well-being pleased me. I even lost weight easily. But then, after succumbing to thoughts like "this is boring, too rigid, or too difficult to maintain," I would fall back to eating almost anything. As I became aware of the rules of these different eating plans, I often thought: "Am I damaging my health by the food I am eating?" The dialogue in my head was characterized by fear and confusion. Which eating plan was I to follow? Which rules should I keep, and which should I break?

Fear acts as a magnet for negative experiences. Focusing too much attention on avoiding something really puts energy into what you don't want. As part of the physical universe we are all subject to the Law of Gravity—"what goes up must come down." So too, we are all subject to the principle of consciousness called the Law of Attraction—"what you think about comes about." Fear, based on negative core beliefs, creates a negative expectation that can become a self-fulfilling prophecy. I knew this intellectually.

But, since I couldn't follow every one of these mutually incompatible diets, what if I was choosing the wrong one? I had too much information, so I had to make choices. The fear of doing the wrong thing attended any course I chose. I had programmed myself for digestive problems, no matter what I ate. *No matter how good the food was, my mental nourishment was rich in anxiety.*

At a workshop I heard myself say, "Something is eating away at me." I wasn't talking about food. But I soon recognized the food-related connection and meaning of my seedthought, "Something is eating away at me." This insight triggered the start of releasing my food fears, my impatience, and my digestive upsets.

All my digestive system beliefs were intertwined. Once I had found the key seedthoughts behind them, they began to unravel, taking many forms. I had been afraid of food and confused about an appropriate nutritional plan for myself. I had past programming related to every type of food I ate—it might be too fatty, or bad for circulation, or hard to digest when eaten in a wrong combination. I was allergic to some foods. I was concerned about preservatives, or that the food was dead and lacking in enzymes. When eating out, I'd worry about improper handling and food spoilage. There were days when everything I ate triggered some fear.

In spite of this, I still loved to eat, but my worrisome thoughts contributed to heightened stress and reduced my sense of well-being. I realized that no matter how good my life got, no matter how peaceful the world became, I would not be at peace until I eliminated my food-related fears. I resolved to let go of fearful food-related thoughts, to eat food, and think thoughts that helped me.

I made a major shift of context. *I pictured my past patterns and unhealthy beliefs being eaten away.* I took that recurrent, unhelpful seedthought, "Something is eating away at me" and turned it against my negative beliefs. In this way, a once-negative thought became a vehicle for my own transformation.

Body as Barometer

The body is a barometer for emotions. You may be unconscious of negativity or upset, but discomfort in your body can point out your emotional distress. Alice Katz, psychotherapist and author of *Compulsive Overeating*, says that "eating is a way we both express and cover up emotion. What we eat, when we eat and why we eat can be related to memories and unconscious beliefs. Memories often trigger the desire to eat.

"One overweight woman client loved pasta. She remembered going to a buffet with her favorite uncle. She took a large plateful of food and then was praised by her family when she went to get more pasta. Another client recalled not being allowed to have candy as a child. Candy was 'forbidden fruit.' For spite, when she got older, she ate candy in great quantities. Eating was her act of defiance: an inappropriate behavior that hurt her as much as anyone."

Many people eat more than necessary when under stress. Alice Katz says, "We use food inappropriately to feed an emotion like loneliness. But loneliness requires people for true comfort." My sister Arlene often says, "I ate my way through Barbara's brain surgery." She uses food to drown her fearful feelings.

A research study by Marvin Acklin and Gene Alexander[31] described in *Brain/Mind Bulletin* found *a clear association between inability to express emotion and a variety of illnesses from gastrointestinal disorders to dermatitis, migraines, and low back pain.*

My friend Jean recently had a ghastly case of twenty-four-hour stomach flu that actually lasted days longer. At the end, she recognized how her sensitivity to stressful feelings had made her more vulnerable to this awful physical upset. She said "I trapped myself in a job with an employer I dislike." By its physical reactions, her body showed Jean how unhappy she was. As soon as she was well enough to work, she left that job.

Lillian, a writer, talked about the intestinal pain she suffered during divorce proceedings. She said "My gut feeling was that there was nothing physically wrong. Still I was in lots of pain. Tests showed I was physically okay. Eventually I realized that I simply 'couldn't stomach' what was going on in this divorce."

Jack, an engineer and a self-improvement junkie, often asked me for self-help advice. Something seemed to be "eating away at him"—he was never satisfied. He spoke of his "gut-level" negative programming, which he had to get rid of. Doctors recently discovered that Jack has a long-standing case of intestinal parasites.

Bernie Siegel, M.D., in *Love, Medicine and Miracles* wrote about a comment from one of his patients after emergency surgery to remove several feet of dead intestine. Siegel really listens to his patients so they often share their true feelings with him. This patient, a Jungian therapist, told Siegel, "I'm glad you're my surgeon, I've been undergoing teaching analysis. I couldn't handle all the shit that was coming up, or digest the crap in my life."[32]

Distressing or negative feelings often arise after we commit ourselves to something that really stretches our abilities. For fifteen years, Henry, a student of mine, was general manager of Jim's profitable wholesale business. When Jim retired, Henry purchased the business using borrowed capital. For the next ten years, Henry struggled to repay the loan and grow the business, working long, hard hours. Managing a business that he owned really stretched his abilities. Henry often said, "Thoughts like, 'Why did I ever buy this business?' keep intruding on my mind. Pressure to repay the loans and keep the business viable don't give me much time or energy for myself. I often feel isolated; there's no one to share this burden. *I feel a hunger and to satisfy it, I eat too much and gain weight.*"

During his free time Henry often complained of headaches and other vague discomforts. His feelings of inadequacy, fear of failure, and general discomfort at being the boss were struggling to be acknowledged. Eventually Henry got the message from his body. He realized that his physical discomforts were telling him to change his attitudes and lifestyle. He alleviated the stress with more rest, relaxation and exercise, and less food. During counseling he realized that he had many choices. He told me, "I could close down the business, or hire someone else to run it, or even sell it. Work was meant to enhance my life, not replace it."

Since Henry was still committed to his business, he hired more people to assist him—a step he had been reluctant to take. He recently said: "I blew it and now I am going to resurrect it." He runs the business now with renewed awareness. He got in touch with the fear and self-doubt that had impeded his ability to make wise choices. Clearing up the emotional stress released the pain, helping his body to feel better. Feeling better helped him to think more clearly. Henry had *digested* his past experiences, *assimilated* information which motivated him to *eliminate* negative thoughts and make many positive changes. His processing continues.

Pow! That Emotion Just Zapped You

A common core belief is that our lives would be great if we could control the external circumstances. That sounds right to many people and yet evidence abounds to the contrary. The true quality of our lives comes from *our internal response.*

For example: one man goes bankrupt and commits suicide, and another learns from the experience and goes on to be successful. One woman gets cancer and bemoans her fate; another uses the experience to make deep inner changes, emerging happier and more peaceful. Some people get yelled at and scream back verbal abuse. Others listen with understanding and compassion, adding peace to a troubled environment. One driver lets you cut in line in front of him, another gives you the finger. These responses come from different inner attitudes, and surely the felt experience of each is different. Each of us determines the quality of our lives through the core beliefs that influence our behavior.

To understand how emotions affect us, it is helpful to understand something about the basic nature of emotion. Emotions are real! These feelings are automatic reactions that reflect our past experiences. Emotions are the primal (original, archetypal, fundamental) instinctive parts of our being. Julia Bondi, author of *Lovelight: Unveiling the Mysteries of Sex and Romance* believes that instinctive emotional reactions to situations help us recognize unconscious core beliefs:

> We have evolved beyond being only instinctual-reactive emotional creatures. We now have the power of thought, a gift from God, to use to harness the energy of our emotions. Emotions as responses are always there, ready to be felt. Experience stimulates them. Thinking about things does too! We react emotionally and the explanation we give ourselves to express and cope with what we instinctively feel, can develop into an unconscious belief. In a sense, we feel the emotion and then attempt to explain away any hurt.

> Because emotions are primal or instinctive, the mind and thought is our way of both getting in touch with them and also directing them appropriately. *Reacting off of emotions, without thinking things through, often leads us to say or do things that we'll later regret.*

Conscious thought helps us deal with our emotions constructively, as long as we don't use our thoughts to judge or deny them. Right thinking allows you to change your inner beliefs, so you can realign them with your emotions in a healthy, useful way.

For example: when I am six months old and hungry, if nobody sticks a bottle or a breast in my mouth, it is primal instinct for me to start yelling to express my emotion. There is no thought there, just the raw emotion. But as I get older I can think about how to satisfy my hunger by doing something appropriate. I can ask Mommy for food or take a cookie from the cookie jar myself.

Thoughts are a bridge to us getting in touch with emotions, because we are no longer just instinctive-emotional people. As we grow up, we become thinking people. By observing and understanding what happens to us, why an experience was necessary, we can recognize unconscious feelings fueling the experience.

For example, baby Jane cries when she sees her doctors. That's a primal, instinctive, emotional reaction on her part—the result of previous, often painful, scary experiences. Doctor visits involve shots, blood work, being poked and even manhandled. As Jane gets older, she may justify her emotional reaction to doctors with the unconscious thought, "Doctors are people that hurt me." On a conscious level she may experience a reluctance to go to doctors and not know why. The unconscious belief (doctors hurt me) will determine her behavior—until she recognizes it. If Jane can understand that the doctor was there for her good, even though the shot felt painful, she can modify her actions based on this understanding.

A more helpful thought would be, "True, those doctors caused me pain when they worked on me, but it was for my own good. I don't need to fear doctors anymore." Her primal emotion of fear is accepted. But the seedthought "doctors hurt me," which was a rigid core belief as an infant, is not valid in the present. Then, she is freed to be helped by her doctors.

Dis-ease is related to an unconscious feeling of "I don't love myself enough" or "I'm not worthwhile." The attendant belief is generally based on forgotten childhood decisions. Perhaps

"Teacher yelled at me. I'm feeling bad so I must be bad." Unconscious belief: "I'm not good enough."

Life experiences trigger your emotional memories. Then your thoughts say, "I can justify feeling this way because of a whole slew of reasons derived from past experiences."

If you don't change the original "I don't love myself" feeling, you justify having and misusing the present-day emotion. You'll take a trip down memory lane reminding yourself of all your past negative beliefs, trapping yourself in a quagmire of unhealthy thoughts. You'll not have a chance to deal with your emotion constructively. You'll say or do something unwise.

In order to change the meaning of the original feeling you must first be conscious of it. Start paying attention to the interior dialogue which validates your feelings. Then you must re-examine the beliefs you've built up from your past experiences with that feeling. You'll need to *recognize your own goodness:* "Even though teacher yelled at me and I felt awful, that doesn't mean I'm bad. I am good enough." The changed dialogue leads to new inner beliefs. You have rid yourself of the primal emotion as a negative force in your life and turned it to your advantage.

Some people develop excessive fears about going to the dentist. Others fear talking in public. They have not come to terms with their original emotional reactions to these events and released their fear. But they can. Once a stressful early event has been uncovered, people are able to bring later learning and adult insight to bear on it. The best way to pacify your emotions is to learn something from them.

Emotions exist. They are always there. Will they run you? Or will you use their energy to build yourself a happy life? The quality of your life is determined more by interior states than by external circumstances. To feel well your emotional as well as your physical digestive system must be in tip-top working order.

Self-Help Experience # 14
Witnessing Practice: Paying Attention to Yourself

Purpose: To expand self-knowledge. Practicing observing yourself as if you were another person leads to greater objectivity and honesty with yourself.

Instructions

1. *Throughout the day observe yourself at regular intervals, while sitting, standing, or walking.* Pretend you are across the room from your body and describe what you see. Don't be discouraged if this is difficult. If you can't see yourself, pretend or imagine you can.

2. Another way to observe yourself is to feel the different parts of your body and *describe to yourself how each part feels.*

Examples:

- I am slouching as I stand.

- There is a pulling sensation in my lower back on the right side.

- I feel a cramp in my abdomen.

- My left arm is itching.

- My eyes are watering.

3. *Notice any thoughts you are having.* You might say, "I have been thinking about..." Then return to your current activity and take your attention off yourself.

4. *Consciously use your mind to tell yourself how you feel physically and emotionally at any given moment.* All of us have experience talking silently to ourselves—that incessant chatter that intrudes on our inner peace. Maybe we have thoughts like, "What if?" or "Why me?" or "How come?" or "What's wrong with him?" Just notice what you are saying to yourself. You don't have to do anything.

Self-Help Experience #15
Questions for Illness

Purpose: To investigate the source of your disease. Your typical ailments can reveal a blueprint in your system. As you observe your recurring symptoms (sore throats, pimples, stomach aches, tumors, sprained ankles), you can uncover the seedthoughts which are triggering these ailments.

Instructions

1. How are you feeling—right now? Describe to yourself the way different parts of your body feel, paying special attention to any uncomfortable sensations. What is your emotional state? Are you happy, sad, angry, bored, excited, curious, interested?

2. Focus your attention on your primary physical complaint. Describe it to yourself.

3. What do you believe is causing your current discomfort?

4. Ask yourself, "What is this dis-ease trying to teach me?"

5. What is going on in your life right now? Recall the past few weeks. What is ahead that you may be dreading or looking forward to?

6. Can you recall a time in the past when you felt this way or experienced similar circumstances?

7. What do you believe would help you to feel better?

It takes practice and self-discipline to understand the message of ill-health. But the reward of a happier, healthier, more contented daily life is worth the time and trouble.

Self-Help Experience #16
Journal Writing

Purpose: To write yourself to greater awareness and self-knowledge

Instructions

1. Record the events of your day and note how you were feeling. Even if you generally have difficulty getting in touch with your feelings, focusing your attention on yourself by keeping a journal will encourage your true feelings to surface. Write at least once each day.

2. List who you saw, where you went, any projects you accomplished, how you generally felt during the day. It is not necessary to write complete sentences. I often use my appointment book to jot down things I want to remember.

3. Once a week, look over your notes and see if you learn anything new about yourself.

For example, to learn how different foods affect you, write what you ate and later note how you felt. Journal keeping can be used to uncover how people, places, or things affect you. When you re-read your journal over several days or weeks, you might discover that whenever you go to a certain place, or see a certain person, you get upset. Often, we know these things subconsciously, but we don't realize the truth consciously until we review our written records. The more you learn about yourself, the easier it will be to make changes.

I need this like a hole in the head
I put my foot in it
I should keep my big mouth shut
Read my lips

Clichés and Body Talk

7

Recently a woman wrote Dear Abby about her beloved boyfriend, saying he does something "that simply kills me." Another common expression is "that person will be the death of me." Why do we talk like that? We mean to express emotion. But using sayings like "that kills me" to express a feeling can be dangerous.

Linda Zelizer is a hypnotist and psychotherapist. One of her male patients had a heart condition. She noted the following interesting behavior: "When he described certain upsetting incidents, he took his right hand and beat his chest, exclaiming, 'That just breaks my heart,' suggesting to his inner mind the image of a broken heart. Upon realizing this, he stopped beating on his chest and using those words. During hypnosis he gave himself positive suggestions such as 'My heart is strong and well.' His heart healed fine."

Phrases like "that breaks my heart" can create an image of a "broken heart" in the subconscious part of the mind which doesn't exercise discrimination or rationality. The seedthought "broken heart" becomes an imaged pattern of beliefs embedded in the body. Frequency of use seems to increase the

the power of the thought to do harm. Language affects us if or when our body translates certain seedthoughts and core beliefs into physical expression.

A Connecticut cardiologist who also has a general practice said, "Patients frequently say 'That breaks my heart' or 'I was heartbroken.' But not just heart patients!" It's reassuring that many people who talk that way don't become cardiac cases. Still, their is a chance that talking that way—using provocative cliché images—can program one for bodily harm. Common sense dictates that prudent behavior would be to eliminate these potentially harmful clichés from our speech. Then *counteract any past programming* by acknowledging "those things in our life that do our heart good."

Burden Seedthoughts

Various bodily sensations like pain and muscle tension can reflect feeling burdened by life. When you feel you have too much to carry, your emotions can translate into a thought like "I can't bear it anymore."

Dr. Jackie Ruzga, a chiropractor practicing in Fairfield, Connecticut, reported: "In the last six months I've had at least a dozen patients who complained, in various words, that they were 'carrying the weight of the world on their shoulders.' Every one of them had shoulder problems. Healing shoulder problems is now a specialty of mine."

Dr. Bob Lang, M.D., is an endocrinologist in Bridgeport, Connecticut. He's also a very good listener. He is currently writing a book about *Healing Conversations*. "The conversations we have with ourselves appear to affect our health. *Illness can result from ineffective conversations*. Back pain, for example, is often associated with someone saying to himself, 'I'm not being supported.' He may not recognize the implications of this thought until I point it out to him during a 'healing conversation.' *Healing is often the result of an effective conversation.*"

The Body Speaks Its Mind

These stories are true examples of people who have discovered messages from their bodies to be messages from their mind and emotions. See if any of these examples ring true for you, although don't forget that each person has his or her own unique signals.

During counseling, Paula, a former student of mine, found evidence of a seedthought that signaled her inner dissatisfaction. Her knee gave her difficulty whenever she had to face something she felt she couldn't bear. She was hanging on to an unhappy marriage and she often said, "I can't bear it." Recognizing the language connection helped Paula choose to exit the unhappy marriage and eventually create a much more satisfying one. If her knee hurts now she knows some inner self-examination is required.

Nina's ankle was sore for two years after a minor injury. She was unable to ice-skate, her favorite recreational activity. During a counseling session, she realized how often she said "I can't stand it." When she realized the connection and stopped feeding herself this negative seedthought, her ankle improved sufficiently for her to resume skating.

Another student, Bob, developed a condition similar to lockjaw after a Novocaine injection. For three months, he could barely open his mouth. After hearing about the language connection Bob told me that he frequently had the thought, "I gotta stop talking." To those people suffering from TMJ—temporomandibular joint dysfunction of the jaw—have you ever berated yourself for talking or eating too much? Have you ever wished you had "kept your big mouth shut?"

The body does not distinguish between our figurative and our literal language; instead it seems to mirror that which we think or speak. Westport, Connecticut psychotherapist and health counselor Roberta Tager provides a personal example: "Recently I was listening to some tapes of a counseling session I had with my supervisor. Self-critically I kept repeating over and over, 'I have to stop talking.' Two days later I lost my voice. Be careful what you say—you may get it!"

Tager has had other experiences of the language connection. She recounted, "Dr. Maxwell headed the admissions committee for his country club. During his term, he frequently said, 'I need this like a hole in the head.' After several years he discovered a growth on his face which left an indentation—a strange growth which looked literally like a 'hole in his head.' The indent, situated on the right side of his face between the temple and the eye, was surgically corrected. A lab report indicated that basal or cancerous cells were completely removed. He no longer uses that cliché."

Sue, a former student, recounted this story: "When I was a little girl my mother and I went on a six-week overseas vacation. As we were leaving for the airport my father told me how much he'd miss me. After that leave-taking, I developed ear infections whenever I traveled by airplane, and I had no idea why. During a self-improvement seminar, I remembered responding to my father's words by thinking, 'I don't want to hear that.' The seed had been planted to 'not hear things' during plane travel. Since uncovering that seedthought and without medical treatment, I am free of the recurrent ear infections. And I travel by plane quite a bit."

Dr. Vincent Scavo, M.D., a Bridgeport ear, nose, and throat specialist, confirms the frequency of cliché talk among his thousands of patients. He said: "You'd be amazed how many patients tell me 'I don't want to hear that! They come to me and I'm their doctor. I shoot straight from the hip. But they don't want to hear when I tell them the truth."

Emily, a professional woman, talked of getting terrible headaches whenever she wore her new glasses. The doctors could find no organic reason for these headaches. She said, "Since I could not see well without my glasses, I went for counseling to see if I could find a psychological reason for my headaches. My therapist asked me, 'What is it you don't want to see?' I realized the truth of that statement. There was something I didn't want to see. I faced the problem and now am able to wear my glasses comfortably. Now I want to see!"

Not everyone has such rapid success. A patient of Linda Zelizer's was having violent arguments with her husband. She realized that her eyesight began to fail when she made the decision, "I don't want to see that." The woman labeled this a coincidence. She believed her failing eyesight was a physical problem only and refused to consider the possibility that it might have another element. When Zelizer tried to make her aware of the mental/emotional component she became angry and resistant, and stopped treatment.

Zelizer said, "I find many people have difficulty with the connection between their body and their words and thoughts. I stress to them that these statements were made *without their awareness* of the possible consequences of such talk. They are then offered the choice of being responsible for themselves or remaining victims. Many, like this woman, seem more comfortable in the role of victim. They refuse to recognize a link between what they think and say, and how they feel."

Another Zelizer patient had lost his voice. During therapy he recalled that after an argument he had had the thought, "Telling people what you think can ruin a relationship." By losing his voice, he insured that he could not say what he thought. He was shocked when he realized he had caused himself laryngitis. He acted on this realization by learning to express himself more appropriately in a caring, yet assertive way. His voice returned in a month.

A female friend was complaining about her pilonidal cyst, a congenital cyst at the base of the spine that can get infected. It can be surgically removed. She told me her cyst got worse each month during her period. I asked her, "Did you ever have the thought that 'having your period was a pain in the ass?'" She gasped as the significance of this idea clicked in for her.

Dr. Carl Gruning, associate professor at SUNY College of Optometry, described a similar case: "One of my patients, a young boy, came to me because he had difficulty concentrating while reading. His ability to focus was impaired and one eye often drifted out—'walleye' in layman's terms. He was referred to me for vision training in the hope of improving his reading ability and concentration. He expressed his problem in these terms, 'My mind drifts off when I am reading.'

"During his vision-training program he learned how to coordinate and focus his eyes and properly integrate the visual system with the rest of his body. His focusing improved markedly after completing the vision therapy. He reads comfortably with improved comprehension. Commenting on the results of his treatment he said, 'My mind rarely drifts off now.'"

Anne, a psychotherapist, took care of her emotionally sick daughter for six months. Later she told me she was angry at her daughter for being sick, but couldn't say anything to her. During that time, a lump developed in Anne's breast. She required a mastectomy to "get it off her chest."

Jane, speaking during a support group meeting, said she often woke up in the morning with her teeth clenched, feeling afraid of something or other. She required lots of dental work. Jane wondered if there was a connection to her oft-repeated statement, "That sets my teeth on edge."

Father Bruce Ritter—the founder of Covenant House, a refuge for kids in trouble—opened a recent fund-raising letter with these words. "If I have to tell the six-kids-that-started-Covenant-House story one more time 'I'm going to blow my brains out.' It's true— the story—every word of it, but I've told it ten thousand times and I'm sick of it." I think Father Ritter's word's are "mind-blowing." I wrote him pointing out the danger of such talk and suggested that he stop writing, thinking, and speaking like that. Apparently, many people had written him, upset at what he'd written. He wrote back that he had merely meant to express emotion. He didn't think then about the literal meaning of his words—though he will from now on.

Mixed Messages

A mixed message is a statement that uses both positive and negative images. Examples are expressions like: "I am pretty upset" or "That was terribly nice." When you hear the words "terrible" and "nice" together, which word do you respond to? Mixed messages can lead to mind-body communication disruptions.

Some words are filled with mixed messages. Awe, for example, is defined by Webster as "fear mingled with admiration or reverence." When someone says "I feel awful" he usually means something negative. But awe-ful in the sense of being filled with awe could be positive. To be in awe of God or beauty is a pleasing idea. But to be in awe is historically an uncomfortable enough experience to lend a negative meaning to the words "I feel aweful."

"I'm sorry," "I feel so bad," "I feel terrible about that." These words are used when apologizing to another, or in expressing sympathy, regret, or remorse. The speaker often doesn't feel bad at all but merely wants to express herself in a forceful way to prove she is genuinely sorry. A sympathizer will say the expected "I feel so badly" and not mean it or really care what's happening to the other person.

Telling yourself or another person that you feel bad can trigger such feelings in body and mind. It's a lie, which is bound to have repercussions: *your words and feelings are in conflict.* "I feel bad," meant as an apology, is an unwise affirmation often perceived by the body as an order for uncomfortable physical feelings. Such common expressions convey to your unconscious mind a set of instructions which can cause disease.

RX: Positive Talk, Positive Thoughts, Positive Attitudes

We can deliberately create helpful seedthoughts. There are phrases common to our language which can help us without our realizing it. For example, Mr. Niles, a former Tager client, was given only a few months to live after being diagnosed as having pancreatic cancer. Two years later, he was doing extremely well. He often says, "I don't let anything bother me anymore." His words indicate a positive attitude which reduces the effect of stressful emotions and supports the efficacy of his chemotherapy treatments. Don't Worry—Be Happy!

Through the enlightened use of language we can often reverse the consequences of prior abuse. Obviously we do use language positively quite often. Notice the balance between your use of positive and negative seedthoughts. It is well worth the effort to prescribe for yourself an increase of positive, health-affirming thoughts and a fast from the negative, diseaseful ones.

Self-Help Experience #17
Verbal Hygiene I

Purpose: To be aware of clichés and other expressions you may use unconsciously

General Instructions

Read through the following lists. Do you use any of these expressions? Ask yourself what emotion you really meant to express. Can you think of a better way to express that feeling? Notice which clichés are most familiar to you. Do they feel right? Perhaps some of them are seedthoughts for you. Ask yourself what effect these sayings might have on your body. Practice verbal hygiene— think before you speak. Cancel or erase those expressions you use which might be unhealthy. Verbal hygiene cleans up your mental act by cleaning up your thoughts and words. Think, speak, and act in ways that prevent disease from occurring physically.

Emotional Phrases, Clichés & Seedthoughts

I get choked up with emotion.
I cried my eyes out.
I'm a nervous wreck.
It blew my mind.
I need this like a hole in the head.
I need to get this out of my head.
I must get this off my chest.
I've got to stop eating.
I let my body go to pot.
I feel stuffed.
I can't stomach him.
I can't digest that.
I got cold feet.
I lost my nerve.
I froze with terror.
I wish I was dead.
I put my foot in it.
I went off my rocker.
I went crazy.
I flipped out.
I nearly died.
I fight:
>   for attention;
>   for what I believe in;
>   for my rights.

I blew:
>   it;
>   my cool;
>   my stack.

I feel:
>   like a square peg in a round hole;
>   all tied up;

I'm a glutton for punishment.
I can't:
  bear it anymore;
  think straight;
  believe it;
  see straight.
I got ambushed (surprised) by a disease, a circumstance.
I'm sorry: I feel so bad;
I feel terrible about that.
I am:
  breaking out;
  burning up;
  itching to get going;
  spaced out;
  uptight;
  sick and tired of;
  sick to death of;
  scared to death of;
  petrified—rigid, frozen, unable to act;
  frozen with fear;
  eaten up with anger;
  in a stew over that;
  heart broken;
  torn apart;
  stiff as a board;
  out of my mind with...(worry, fear, grief);
  in a dead-end situation;
  dead on my feet;
  not good enough;
  too good for you;
  at the boiling point;
  overcome with emotion.
I am dying to:
  retire;
  do that;
  get that;
  see that
  ...and so on.

That:

> was a pain in the neck;
> gives me a headache;
> breaks my heart;
> drives me crazy;
> will give me a heart attack;
> will be the death of me;
> makes my blood boil;
> tears my guts apart;
> rips me apart;
> just kills me;
> makes me sick to my stomach;
> sets my teeth on edge;
> makes my skin crawl;
> is hard to swallow;
> weighs on me;
> is nerve wracking;
> is a bitter pill to swallow.

There's a knot in my stomach.
Something is eating away at me.
My heart feels shut down.
My mind drifts off.
My feet are killing me.
It is:

> eating at my gut;
> a pain in the ass;
> just my luck;
> in my blood.

My nerves are raw.
What an unnerving experience.
The crisis reached a head.

Self-Help Experience #18
Verbal Hygiene II–Group Seedthoughts

Purpose: To uncover some prejudices and widely held beliefs

The purpose of these lists is to assist you in observing your mind. Your thoughts and words are indicative of your beliefs. Then consciously decide: "Are these ideas really true for me? Do I want to hold on to these beliefs?" Some of these are clichés, some are seedthoughts, and some are not. But all represent a definite set of beliefs held by various groups of people. Sometimes in your conscious mind you may reject an idea. But if you have heard it often enough, any of the following ideas may actually be part of the fabric of your unconscious belief system. You could be affected by them without realizing it. Truly, the examined life is most worth living.

Which of the following statements do you have lurking in the depths of your mind, like time bombs or mines waiting to explode? Some of them like "Honesty is the best policy" might even be good for you. But let it be your conscious choice now to keep them.

Health-related Beliefs:

> Old age brings illness.
>
> Only the good die young.
>
> Cancer, stroke, or heart disease cause death.
>
> AIDS is always fatal.
>
> Disease attacks regularly through life. There is little that can be done about it. Sickness is inevitable.
>
> That disease (cancer, stroke etc.) runs in my family.
>
> That was the straw that broke the camel's back.
>
> Without medicine that (disease) can't improve.
>
> You must move your bowels once a day.
>
> I'll die at the same age as my parents.
>
> No pain no gain.
>
> An apple a day keeps the doctor away.
>
> Grin and bear it.
>
> Blow a gasket.
>
> Blow my brains out.
>
> Roll over and play dead.
>
> I should have my head examined.
>
> I did it just for the hell of it.
>
> I need to 'spill my guts.'
>
> Cry yourself to death; laugh yourself to health.
>
> Stress:
>> can kill you;
>>
>> is bad for you;
>>
>> is good for you.
>
> I was caught off guard.
>
> Ignorance is/is not bliss.
>
> What you don't know won't hurt you.

Prosperity, Work, and Sex-related Beliefs:

> Money is power.
> You need to have money to make money.
> More of "anything" is better. Less is more.
> Men are more interested in sex than women.
> All men care about is sex.
> Women take forever to come.
> Women use sex to "control" men.
> Men use money to "control" women.
> What you resist persists.
> Seeing is believing.
> What you sow you reap.
> What goes around, comes around.
> Honesty is the best policy.
> When the going gets tough, the tough get going.
> Better late than never.
> You just can't win.
> It's a no-win situation.
> A stitch in time saves nine.
> I'll be the first one laid off, you wait and see.
> It always happens to me.

Eating Metaphors—Food for Thought:

> Now you're cooking.
> Feed your mind.
> Hungry for sex.
> Eat your words.
> Chew on it.
> Swallow your pride.
> You're full of it.
> That has a bite to it.
> Eating:
>> too much is bad;
>> too little is bad.

Superstitious Beliefs—Common Sayings:

> Good things always come with bad.
> Things, good or bad, happen in threes.
> Friday the 13th is a bad luck day.

Don't walk under a ladder.

Step on a crack, break my back.

Don't let a black cat cross your path.

Garlic around the neck wards off evil.

Cross your heart and hope to die.

Cross your fingers—to allow you to lie.

Cross your fingers—for good luck.

See a penny pick it up, all day long you'll have good luck.

Let sleeping dogs lie.

Relationship-related Beliefs:

Being competitive brings out the beast in us. Being cooperative brings out the best in us.

Revenge is sweet.

Change is easier if not changing carries a price.

Girls are better at....

Boys are better at....

Girls drive me crazy.

Boys drive me crazy.

Good guys finish last.

If you don't have something nice to say, don't say it.

Why is everybody always picking on me?

Never trust:

> a woman;

> a man.

Never trust anyone:

> over thirty;

> under thirty.

There is something inherently wrong with everyone (the biblical concept of original sin).

Racial Stereotypes:

Practically every racial and religious group is subject to prejudices against them. Following are some of the hundreds of racial and ethnic beliefs. Notice how harmful these stereotypical ideas can be to peaceful world relations. Which of these group prejudices are familiar? Do you believe them?

Jews are money hungry.

Arabs lie and cheat.

Moslems are fanatics.

Christians are fanatics.

Black is:
    beautiful;
    ugly.
They are: good dancers; great athletes; poor students.
English are cold.
Irish drink a lot.
The luck of the Irish.
Never trust: a Frenchman; a German.
You can't trust the Russians.
Americans are loud and brash.
Orientals are: frugal; hard working; smart; untrustworthy; inscrutable.
Mexicans are dumb, lazy.
Cubans are tough.
Italians are: mafia crooks; over-sexed.
They...(any group but your own)...aren't as good, smart, nice etc. as we (your group) are.

Self-Help Experience #19
Verbal Hygiene III—Words That Wound & Words That Heal

Purpose: To recognize more damaging and helpful ways of speaking and thinking

    Knock 'em dead.
    Read it and weep.
    You are:
        not good enough for me;
        too good for me.
        an accident waiting to happen;
        a walking time bomb (often said prior to heart attack or stroke);
        a jerk, dumb, stupid, an idiot,
        no good;
        so kind;
        a glutton for punishment;
        too hard on yourself;
        so beautiful;
        good as gold;
        smart as a whip;
        thick-skinned;
        thin-skinned;

> tight-lipped;
>> a sight for sore eyes.

It's good to see you.
Good for you.
Be careful or:
> you'll fall;
> catch cold;
> …and so on.

Swallow your feelings when...
Drown your sorrows.
It does my heart good when...
Smile and the world smiles with you.
Share and share alike.
It never hurts to be nice.
Read my lips.
Eat your heart out!
Bite your tongue!
It's just not fair!
You will never amount to anything.
Why did I say that?
Swallow your pride.
I couldn't do that.
I'm afraid not.
I hate you.
I love you.
If only..!
What if...?
Why me...?
Keep on keeping on.
If at first you don't succeed, try, try again.
When the going gets tough, the tough get going.
You're not yourself today. You don't look good.
You look:
> tired;
> sick;
> wonderful;
> handsome;
> beautiful.

It ain't over 'till the fat lady sings.

Make the best of it.

Make the most of it.

Expect the best. Prepare for the worst.

This too shall pass!

Move traffic in the direction it's going.

Out of the mouths of babes often comes wisdom.

An ounce of prevention is worth a pound of cure.

Count your blessings.

Every day in every way I'm getting better and better.

I wish you many blessings.

Self-Help Experience #20
Releasing Painful Emotion

Purpose: To get over hurt feelings and prevent the need to get a physical illness to express your emotion

Instructions

1. Acknowledge your hurt, but don't dwell on it. The longer you dwell on an emotion, the more at home you feel, and the more likely you are to induce illness.

2. Express your hurt feelings in positive ways, like crying or talking it out.

3. Find ways to nurture yourself with positive activities like exercising, taking a bath, or having a massage.

4. Remove negative thoughts by replacing them with more positive ones. Think something as simple as, "It does my heart good to see a rainbow, or listen to music, or eat a good meal (or whatever you like to do)." Even if you are deeply unhappy you can find something that makes you feel good.

5. If you find yourself dwelling in self-pity, whether justified or not, remembering other people in worse circumstances is sometimes helpful.

You see what you believe.
It never rains but it pours.
I should live so long.

Perceptions About Health and Disease

8

Our beliefs about the way things are shape the way we see things. The notion that prophecy can be self-fulfilling has some scientific truth. Researchers in perception have demonstrated that we often see what we expect to see, hear what we expect to hear, and feel what we expect to feel. Daily news stories provide examples of this. We may all hear the same words or read the same story, but how we interpret it, what it means to us, comes from our underlying beliefs. Your race, nationality, cultural, political and religious beliefs predispose how you will view a given event. Consider Ollie North of Iran-Contra fame: Is he traitor or patriot? Your answer to this question depends on what you believe about a whole variety of issues. Most conservatives view North as a hero and most liberals see him as a traitor.

When what we believe comes to pass, that reinforces our core belief. Often what we believe will be true to us, precisely because we believe it! In order to experience a shift in attitude, we must be open-minded enough to view new evidence and change our inner beliefs. To the extent that we are aware of our beliefs and willing to suspend them, we can learn to

95

suspend them, we can learn to view any event objectively.

Scientists are supposed to be searching for totally objective truths. Yet they are now beginning to realize that they design instruments and experiments in order to find certain expected effects. In other words, what they expect to find conditions the way they search for it. They then often find what they are looking for, since all their efforts have been directed to this end. The way we believe the world is, is the way we create it.

We actually perceive things selectively, not noticing all that enters our field of attention. To a couch potato, a switched-on TV muffles the outside world. A child, engrossed in play, won't hear his mother call him for dinner. A cat stalking a mouse does not hear sounds it could not miss before the mouse appeared. Indeed, as Daniel Goleman Ph.D. says in *Vital Lies, Simple Truths,* "perhaps the most crucial act of perception is in making the decision as to what will and will not enter awareness. This filtering is carried out before anything reaches awareness; the decision itself is made outside awareness."[33]

You don't just see with your eyes and hear with your ears. You see and hear with your mind and brain. This lack of attention to new ideas and information often prevents people from recognizing and ultimately changing unhealthy beliefs.

When I am afraid because I believe I may have an illness, my thoughts put my body into a state of agitation and unrest, conditions that support the appearance of disease. But, if I believe I am healthy, I will find evidence to support that belief. I will feel more relaxed, becoming the healthy person that I believe in. Disease is allowed by the mind, even if not necessarily caused by it. Bodily conditions and seedthoughts both reflect our beliefs. In a sense, the body is a "solidified" version of the mind! Edgar Cayce, the great twentieth-century mystic and healer summed it up by saying, "Thoughts are things and mind is the builder."

Beliefs and The Immune System

How we perceive our world appears to affect our immunity to disease. Dr. Paul Pearsall relates that "Dr. Steven Locke at Harvard University Medical School found that natural killer-cell activity is diminished, not by severe changes or stressors in the life of healthy human volunteers, but by people's interpretations of stress: whether or not they see themselves as able to deal effectively with the stress that they are experiencing. It was as if immune cells behaved as confidently as the thinker in which the cells circulate. Dr. Steven Maier and associates, a University of Colorado research team, wondered whether aspects of the immune system would be responsive to 'perception'—the way the brain deals with our world. They found, in their studies with rats and killer cell effectiveness, that *not being in control* results in less effectiveness."[34]

Dr. Sandra Levy found that women treated for breast cancer show more effective killer cell activity if they are agitated than if they are resigned to their fate. Clearly, how we think and feel about what happens to us has a direct effect on our health. Believe in the strength of your body and it will reward you.

Pearsall also states, "It is not just stress or life pressures that affect our immunoefficiency, but our perceptions of our world as well....Researchers now know that cells within the immune system and within the brain itself have receptors on them that allow for interaction between the immune system and the brain. Every thought and every feeling we have alters the immune system, and every challenge to the immune system alters the way we think and feel."[35]

Flexible Thinking Creates Flexible Bodies

Many years ago, psychotherapist Roberta Tager was diagnosed as having multiple sclerosis, or MS, a degenerative disease of the central nervous system in which hardening of tissue occurs. She describes her experience this way:

> I saw some of the subconscious patterns that had shaped me, causing my disease. My thinking was rigid; my focus on the way to do most things was narrow. I wasn't aware that there were options in *any* situation.
>
> When I was first sick, something as mundane as being locked out of my house threw me off balance. If an obstacle arose I was almost *paralyzed, I was frozen in place.* My emotional energy would build up as I needed to find a solution. When none presented itself I felt my energy turn in on me. I felt frazzled! The energy going down my spine burned. There was no place for this energy to go, no way for

me to use it. I believe that had a literal effect on my nervous system: frazzling and frying the nerves, and triggering my MS symptoms. Damaged nerves are less effective at transmitting movement messages to the muscles. I now understand that excess energy needs to be released in harmless ways, not turned in upon the host vehicle. The body is not designed to store excess energy, stress or emotion without eventually leading to breakdown and disease.

Frozen thought patterns prevented my energy from being used in more creative ways. I believed life was filled with dead ends. Rigid in my thinking and often feeling paralyzed, I could not have verbalized these feelings at that time. But now I see the language connections that fueled these patterns and created my diseased body. MS is a disease with rigidity in the musculature and sometimes paralysis. For some people MS does become a dead end.

My initial reaction to the diagnosis of MS was total fear. Fear of being crippled, paralyzed or dying an early death is a potent force. However I chose another path. I reconnected with my inner voice. It led me to release my fear of MS—and a reduction of the symptoms ensued. To all intents and purposes I have been healed, being free of signs of the disease for more than twenty years. Visualization, relaxation, vitamin therapy and mind control were part of the healing process along with my inner work: changing beliefs and opening myself to my own creativity.

A lot of mental energy fed Roberta's seedthoughts and she manifested a serious physical disorder. For some people, underlying rigidity of beliefs might result in an unyielding and rigid body with other disease labels. In her case the rigid attitudes began to manifest in a process called multiple sclerosis, which could have led eventually to a total inability to act. She woke up in time.

It would be wrong to conclude from Roberta's case that all cases of MS arise from rigid attitudes. That is just one possible language connection. Nor will all people with rigid attitudes develop a major disease. Some people might just have a less flexible body. The desirable state is an ability to be open and flexible in mind and body, when such flexibility is necessary, and firm when that is required.

Your personality and your thought processes can increase or decrease your potential for contracting a disease related to the immune system. George F. Solomon, M.D., Professor of Psychiatry at UCLA, studied female patients with rheumatoid arthritis—a disease that results from aberrant immune function. They "show more masochism, self-sacrifice, denial of hostility, compliance-subservience, depression and sensitivity to anger than their healthy sisters, and are described as always having been nervous, tense, worried, highly strung, moody individuals."[36] He notes that physically healthy relatives with rheumatoid factor—which may predispose them to developing the disease—appear to be psychologically healthier as well. It seems that a "combination of physical predisposition and a breakdown of psychological defenses leads to manifest disease." One of the origins of the idea of a self-fulfilling prophecy might thus be the reality that our bodies fulfill the prophecies our minds make up.

Hypnosis and Beliefs

Hypnotherapist Linda Zelizer says "Sometimes people come for hypnosis to change a specific habit and a deeper issue surfaces. Although they want to change the habit at one level, they first must be willing to deal with their beliefs at a deeper level. They may have some emotional investment in *not* solving the problem. I have encountered many cases in which hypnosis uncovered deeper issues that had to be dealt with in order to release the unwanted condition. Amongst them are these:

- John Kaiser wanted to stop smoking because of an advanced case of emphysema. However, at a primitive level he believed that if he stopped smoking he would be acquiescing to the demands of his wife and mother, both of whom constantly kept after him to quit smoking. Continuing to smoke had become a symbol of rebellion and freedom on a subconscious level.

- Ann Carey had a heart condition and was afraid of dying. She was very overweight, and worried about illnesses associated with this condition. She often thought while she ate: 'What's the use? I don't care if I die!' In a sense she was slowly killing herself. She acknowledged that below the level of her surface symptoms, a part of her was depressed and wanted to die.

• Georgina Roberts was a young woman who wanted to lose weight but was terrified of being thin. She equated being thin with being sexually attractive. She had been molested by an uncle as a young girl. He frequently told her he couldn't resist her because she had such a lovely body.

These cases illustrate how core beliefs affect surface issues and might prevent them from being dealt with. When you get in touch with the underlying beliefs, you cope better with the feelings they engender. You can consciously decide for yourself whether any deeply held belief is still true or useful to you.

John might harmonize his fear of being controlled with his desire to live and decide to stop smoking in spite of the power struggle with the women in his life. He might tell himself, "They aren't trying to control me, they are sharing their love for me. They just want me to live." Ann should explore the roots of her depression and then decide if death is what she wants. Coming to grips with the depression will free her to deal with her weight and illness anxieties. Georgina must recognize and accept her feelings related to being molested and then ask herself: "Do I want that awful incident to rule my life? Do I have to be fat to protect myself from men?"

There are many other examples of self-fulfilling prophecies. Consider the explanation that some women offer for irritability at a certain time each month. Right before menstruation the dreaded "pre-menstrual tension" evokes phrases such as "I expect my period any minute now." During menstruation women often say "Well, I have my period," words meant to excuse any untoward behavior. This language reflects a widely held belief that when women are in the menstrual part of their monthly cycle, they don't act rationally and they should be excused for their behavior then.

The physical changes that occur monthly are real and premenstrual tension is often accompanied by horrendous behavior. But how much do our words affect the experience? Are they cause or effect? Which comes first: the experience or the belief? When women accept as inevitable the condition called premenstrual tension, they doom themselves to repeating it. A better approach is to look for thoughts contributing to or triggering it, in addition to using the many medical techniques now available to help manage this condition.

If we see menstruation as a time when our negative programming is closer to the surface, we can use this time of the month as an opportunity to recognize and then alter such programming. Menstruation brings things that are normally buried out into the open, where they can be seen on a conscious level, and so healed.

I'm Gonna *Live* Till I Die!

My friend Debby told me about her Uncle Harry. He frequently said "I'm never going to live to be fifty," indicative of his lifelong belief that he would die before his fiftieth birthday. During routine gall bladder surgery the day before his fiftieth birthday, Uncle Harry died on the operating table.

It has been widely reported that Elvis Presley believed that older performers like Bing Crosby and Rudy Vallee had degenerated into caricatures of themselves in their primes, doing the same things they'd done years before. His seedthought, "I'll never let that happen to me." He died at age forty-two, never having had the chance to age more gracefully.

When you expect to feel good, your positive attitude helps create it, no matter what the circumstances. Not always, but usually, expecting the best paves the way for the best to occur. To expect the worst paves the way for the worst to be fulfilled. The notion behind a self-fulfilling prophecy is the concept that *what we believe is what comes to pass*. Self-awareness and honest self-evaluation, bringing your core beliefs to the surface, are keys to a healthy life.

Self-Help Experience #21
I Believe...

Purpose: To uncover your beliefs

Make a list. Start with the statement,"I believe..." You fill in the blanks. Work on your list a few minutes a day. You will soon have a rather long list. Keep a pencil beside your bed. I often awake at night with another belief to include on my list.

Sample Belief Statements

Which, if any, of these statements are true about you?

A. I am lovable and kind.

A. My body feels good enough.

A. I think healthy thoughts.

A. I think for myself.

A. I am committed to getting well.

A. People often help me.

A. There is a higher power looking after me.

B. I am selfish and self-centered.

B. I often feel bad.

B. I often think negatively.

B. I let the doctor decide.

B. I'll never get well.

B. People are out to get me.

B. I'm alone in a hostile world.

By now you probably get the idea and can create your own set of questions to uncover your beliefs.

Self-Help Experience #22
Making Believe

Purpose: To practice changing your current circumstances by directing your mind; using thought power to generate better physical and emotional health

I've imagined getting things all my life. Often, like most of us, I have imagined the worst outcome. Now, I use imagination with greater awareness of my mental power. When I realize that I am picturing the worst, I cancel the negative scenario and replace it with a more desirable one. This process works well for me.

For example, two years after my brain surgery, I was given a surgical option for improving my voice by injecting a surgically-used form of teflon into my paralyzed vocal cord. This would expand and stiffen the paralyzed left cord, allowing the right working cord to reach and vibrate against it, improving the quality of my voice. But some part of me didn't like the idea of using teflon. While searching for the right doctor to help me, I frequently wished there were some other way to move the cords closer together. I often thought, "Why can't they just put something near my paralyzed cord in order to move it over so the good one can reach it."

Imagine my astonishment when I was told about a new operation, developed in Japan, that uses a small piece of plastic to press the paralyzed cord permanently closer to the working one. The operation was performed and my voice improved.

You can make believe to encourage your chances of achieving any desired result. While completing this manuscript and waiting for acceptance by a publisher, I often imagined myself receiving a phone call from the publisher telling me, "I loved your book and want to publish it." I made up details of the conversation and even placed a bottle of champagne in my refrigerator to celebrate when I received the call. Since you are reading it now, you know I was successful.

Instructions

Think of a situation in your life that is consistently negative; one you want to change. Visualize the outcome you want. For example: If you want to lose weight, see yourself thin. Pretend you are eating less of the fattening foods. Compliment yourself for choosing to eat wisely. Make believe you are exercising more. Make up or imagine a scenario that will encourage modification of your former fat-inducing behavior. If you begin to eat less food and exercise more, you will certainly lose weight.

When you make believe, you are *pretending* something is so. Often that will motivate you to enact new behaviors and attitudes that are necessary to success. Making believe is a way to make real consciously chosen healthy beliefs. The positive thoughts and feelings generated will have a positive physiological effect on you. You will be encouraged to think and act differently.

You can also imagine a desired outcome over which you don't appear to have any control. Often, you will generate the desired result anyway, like my vocal cord enhancement surgery. A classic example happens when you drive to a place where parking is usually difficult. Somehow, if I expect to get a parking space I do. Some people call this sort of thing coincidence. But, expectation does seem to shape reality.

Self-Help Experience #23
Take a Stand

Purpose: To practice speaking in a creative, self-generating way to achieve results. You take a stand by saying something is so and committing to it through your words and thoughts. You aren't lying, you are creating anew, using your will and imagination to pretend and make believe until you alter your reality. You are living in faith rather than in circumstances.

1. Choose a situation that you desire to change, even a seemingly hopeless one. Declare your stand.

2. Notice any block to achieving your result. Do what you can to remove it. There may be nothing you can do.

3. Express confidence in the final outcome, often and aloud. Ask someone to agree that you will achieve your desired result.

4. Remove your attention from current circumstances. Focus instead on the desired end result.

5. Recognize that there is a higher power at work in your life. So, give thanks for any signs of progress.

6. If it doesn't work out as you desired, recognize and accept that some things just aren't meant to be. Learn something from the experience. Don't just berate yourself.

Self-Help Experience #24
Recognizing and Re-Thinking Unhelpful Thoughts

Purpose: To practice releasing worries by recognizing and changing seedthoughts. This exercise is useful for any upset including health concerns, money and business worries or even fear of failure.

1. *Separate the situation from the emotion.* What emotion are you feeling related to the upsetting situation? Is it anger, fear, frustration, envy, or something else?

2. *Notice your thoughts:* What are you telling yourself related to the upset?

3. *Talk about your thoughts* with someone who can be trusted to help you transform any negative belief into a more helpful seedthought. Don't tell anyone who is going to agree with your negative self-judgment.

4. *Create a new, more positive seedthought.* For example, if you are worried about money say, "Money does not slip through my fingers, since I am so cautious. So even though my worries cost me emotionally, they have helped keep my business solvent. I admire myself for this." This sort of statement will help you see your fears in a positive, more useful context. So find a way of recontextualizing your fears.

5. Following are *sample seedthoughts* that you can adapt to your situation.

    I am confident and make decisions quickly and easily.

    I handle my financial responsibilities with pleasure.

    I'm a strong decisive leader and manager.

    I have as much money as I need to pay all my bills on time.

Self-Help Experience #25
Positive Expectations in Negative Situations

Purpose: How many times have you said, "I am getting a cold" or "I am going to be sick"? Were you right? This exercise is designed to help you stop an illness in its tracks; to alter your unhealthy expectations.

Picture another possibility. Could you allow yourself to be wrong and not fulfill your belief? Wouldn't it be wonderful to stay healthy because you *stop affirming your belief* in a future illness? You can take precautions if you recognize signs that might mean an impending cold. These could include resting more, taking extra Vitamin C and zinc, avoiding dairy products for a time, gargling, taking a hot bath. Do whatever you believe might help you avoid a cold, but don't assume that the cold is inevitable. There is a fine line between creating ill-health by ignoring warning signals and fooling yourself into creating better health.

Instructions

1. Use this the next time you think you are getting some particular ailment such as a cold, sore throat, headache, upset stomach, or backache.

2. First, ask yourself if you need time off from your usual activities. Then give yourself permission to take that time, so you won't need an illness to get a day off. Take a wellness break instead. Do you need solitude or company? Take steps to fill that need without getting ill.

3. Describe to yourself how the ailment you're thinking about makes you feel. Be specific. Do whatever you need to do for your body and for your emotions to avoid this ailment.

4. Find a more favorable way of speaking about how you feel. Instead of "I am getting a cold," tell yourself, "My body is signalling me. I need some free time. I will listen to my body and take a wellness break." Take a stand for good health and you can often generate it.

5. In the event that you do get sick, take care of your body using any physical remedies you know to be helpful. Mend your mind and emotions by imagining and expecting a quick, favorable outcome, a return to health.

Reversing an unwanted situation or ailment is often a slow, difficult thing to do. Sometimes it may be necessary for the process to persist in order for you to learn something from the experience. There is no need for guilt or believing you haven't done it right. Never be hard on yourself if an exercise doesn't seem to work for you. Be easy on yourself. If it doesn't work for you, it's often for the best.

See no evil, hear no evil, speak no evil
What you don't know won't hurt you
You're driving me crazy

Mental Projection
and Expectations

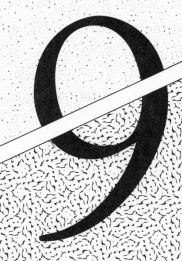

By now it should be clear that your words and thoughts can affect you. But your words and thoughts also influence others, just as theirs affect you. You know the power of a smile or a few kind words to brighten someone else's day. The loving words of a friend can help you feel less stressed. Compare that feeling to the effect angry words have on you. The words and thoughts of others affect you more than you realize. Their destructive potential is even more serious in this nuclear age. We each must be aware of what we are thinking so that our resulting words and actions will add health, love, harmony, and peace to planet Earth.

Doctors' words influence us because we tend to endow physicians with powers of knowing and healing. This is fine when they give reassurance or necessary medical advice. But there are times when doctors' words can needlessly alarm patients with negative messages. Even bad news ought to be given in a positive light.

During a workshop led by Dr. Bernie Siegel, he talked about the role of the physician in chemotherapy. Traditionally, cancer specialists warn patients to expect the unpleasant side effects of chemotherapy, including nausea and vomiting. Some prepare the patient to cope by giving instructions like, "Keep a pail beside your bed." This may be helpful advice, but it tends to generate a hypnotic expectation on the part of the patient. Often these patients fulfill the doctors' expectations by suffering side effects.

But nausea and vomiting are not the inevitable effects of chemotherapy. Quite the contrary, many of Dr. Siegel's patients do not experience any ill effects. Since he recognizes that the subconscious mind is a strong force in healing, he doesn't prepare his patients for suffering after their treatment. Rather, he helps them to see their treatment as a therapy which they have chosen. Those patients who recognize this choice often have less difficulty.

One patient Siegel spoke about during his workshop refused chemotherapy and radiation treatment because she viewed them as poisons—as intrusive techniques with dangerous side effects. With that attitude, she probably would have problems using the techniques, no matter how valuable they might have been. Gradually, however, she altered her thinking until she recognized radiation and chemotherapy as positive forms of energy which could help her to heal. Changing her beliefs allowed her to accept these treatments into her body with peace of mind. When she finally chose to use radiation and chemotherapy, her experience was very positive. While her body repaired itself, she felt fine, even continuing to work during the course of treatment.

Self-Fulfilling Prophecies

In describing a treatment, your doctor probably disclosed its potential side effects. I favor this as a usual procedure, especially when substantial risks are involved. These symptoms would otherwise catch you unawares and generate uncertainty and fear. But there is a real possibility that you will take your doctor's words too seriously and bring on the very side effect that you would want to avoid. You can prevent this by being aware of the effect of negative expectations and by using positive thinking.

Siegel recounts: "If I give you an injection of saline solution and say, 'Here's chemotherapy, Phil; your hair is going to fall out.' thirty percent of men will have their hair fall out." One-third of women, too, receiving placebos instead of chemotherapy, will lose their hair.

Patients sometimes suffer from side effects without ever having been warned. So when a drug seems appropriate, the doctor faces a dilemma: "How do I keep the patient informed while still being positive?" One solution is to inform the patient within a framework of hope. The doctor might say, for example, "Some people have experienced nausea after chemotherapy, but more and more people are avoiding this unpleasant aftereffect. I suspect you will be one of them."

Patients, too, are responsible and should only accept treatments they feel good about and have faith in. We have to trust both ourselves and our doctors for a treatment to succeed. Many patients are able to heal themselves and prevent or minimize the side effects of their treatment by using visualization (positive imagining) or affirmations (positive phrases) to create a mental picture of the most desired outcome.

Healing Conversations

Reducing panic—an important first step in a patient's recovery—is another way that the words of others can affect us. Panic arises from belief in a feared outcome. Hope is belief in a desired outcome. In a well-known story recounted in *The Healing Heart,* Norman Cousins spoke reassuringly to a man felled by a probable heart attack on a golf course. The man's panic subsided as he accepted Cousins's hope-filled words. Within a minute his heartbeat was slower and more regular; his color returned; he looked around and showed interest in his treatment.[37]

Dr. Jackie Ruzga was an emergency room staff nurse before completing her chiropractic studies. She reports:

> When a patient came in with an emergency condition—such as cardiac arrest or acute diabetic shock—a primary nursing goal was to get the patient to feel secure, comfortable, and free of panic. This agitated fear causes hyperventilation which leads to higher than normal heart rate and depletion of oxygen in the body. On more than one occasion I saw evidence of the positive effect of a loving touch and a few well-chosen, hope-filled words. 'Everything is under control. You'll be fine.'

One patient with arrhythmia—abnormal heart rate—was in a highly agitated state. I put my hand on his back and spoke reassuringly to him. His heart rate normalized almost immediately. A young man, a victim of a motorcycle accident, was in shock, bleeding from multiple wounds. Calming the patient is an important part of slowing down bleeding. After reassurance, this man was sufficiently relaxed to have a compound fracture set without anesthesia.

The nurse is like a surrogate mother. By touching and talking she reassures her patients, which helps to keep them alive. One man, about to undergo diagnostic tests, said he was 'frightened to death' of all the high-tech equipment around him. After some reassuring words of explanation, he went through the studies without any further problems.

Patients need to be talked to and touched, since they often feel isolated and alone. That's why the sponge bath is such an important part of good nursing care. This warm communication between nurse and patient helps to relieve anxieties, because it tells the patient that someone cares about them; they are not alone in their time of need.

Even unconscious patients need reassurance. Bernie Siegel writes, "In the operating room I'm constantly communicating with patients about what is happening, and I've found that this can make the difference between life and death. Talking to patients who are having cardiac irregularities during surgery can reverse the irregularities or slow a rapid pulse."[38] Even unconscious patients respond to words of hope and love.

Surgeons have in the past believed that patients under anesthesia don't hear or remember what happened in the operating room. Daniel Goleman describes research at a Chicago Hospital that tested the effects of a message on patients undergoing back surgery.[39] While fully anesthetized these patients were given a suggestion to help them avoid the common postoperative complication of inability to urinate, which then requires catheterization to remove their urine. Not a single patient receiving the suggestion during surgery required catheterization. Of those in a control group who heard no suggestion during surgery, more than half did require catheterization. Whether you remember hearing them or not, other people's words can affect you.

Expectations

Scary information about a disease from the media, the medical profession, and friends can influence people to hold beliefs and fears that negatively affect the outcome of the disease. You get more upset if you *expect* the dire outcome. Roberta Tager says, "All illness is a group of symptoms that happen to be present at the time of diagnosis. If you name the symptoms you give power to them and they are more likely to stay with you because now you have a documented illness in which you believe. Naming can be helpful to healing by pointing to the appropriate treatment or harmful if it fosters negative expectations and an attitude of hopelessness."

Multiple Sclerosis is a diagnosis that often provokes terror. Tager considers herself fortunate that so little was known about MS when she was diagnosed in 1963, as she had less negative information to dwell on. She found her own way. Cancer is another diagnosis that still provokes terror. Cancer represents suffering, even a death sentence, though treatments and survival rates for cancer keep improving. Far from being a death sentence, cancer often gives people a chance to make positive lifestyle changes—learning to live life more fully, productively, lovingly, and joyfully. Illness can be a powerful motivating force. It presents an opportunity for learning and personal growth, since humans often grow through the challenge of adversity.

Bernie Siegel and others often talk about the gift of an illness. Learning to give and receive love is frequently an unexpected positive side effect of some illnesses. I can confirm this from my experience during brain surgery. I felt the unconditional love of my family.

The skillful physician communicates truthful information about your condition while maintaining optimism; something difficult to do if the doctor believes your disease is a hopeless condition. No condition, however, is truly hopeless until you are dead.

Erik Esselstyn, formerly a college dean, now a therapist, has survived bile duct cancer for over 12 years. In discussing the power of hope he says, "When I left the hospital following surgery, chemotherapy and radiation were ruled out, being ineffective in this type of cancer. But, the surgeon gave me hope when he said, 'Come back and see me in five years.'

"I reasoned, 'The doctor expects me to live if he doesn't want to see me for five years. He has set a long-term goal—way out in the future. I'll shoot for that mark.' Hope is a potent force in the healing process, a force that this capable doctor wisely activated. I remain grateful to him. Though uncertain then about my survival, I was determined to do everything possible to aid my complete healing."

Many patients respond to expectations when given pills with no intrinsic healing power, especially if they believe the pills will help them. This placebo effect is an example of a self-fulfilling prophecy. Studies of the placebo effect demonstrate the power of belief and faith in the healing process. Since people often are unaware of their true beliefs, many heal whether they think they believe in the treatment or not.

The classic, oft-recounted case demonstrating the power of expectation in healing involved a male, advanced cancer patient of psychologist Dr. Bruno Klopfer. Krebiozen, a now-discredited drug then receiving widespread acclaim, was being tested at the clinic where the man was a patient. After begging for the treatment, he was given one injection. Shortly after receiving the drug, the patient's cancerous growths "melted like snowballs" apparently freeing him from the disease. Treatment was continued with the drug three times a week till the patient was discharged.

Shortly thereafter, news spread that the drug was worthless. After hearing the news and losing hope, this patient's tumors promptly recurred.

Klopfer, recognizing the powerful effect of his patient's belief system, gave him new hope when he told him that he would give him a specially prepared, more active form of the drug. For this treatment, administered with much fanfare, Klopfer, in fact, used a fresh water placebo. The tumors again melted away, more dramatically than before. The water injections were continued since they worked such wonders, and the patient remained symptom-free for a time. Several months later definitive studies were published showing beyond a doubt that Krebiozen was worthless. Upon learning of this, the man's tumors reappeared, and he soon died.

Ronald Glasser, M.D., in The *Body Is The Hero,* reports on "a paper published in the early thirties in the *Journal of The American Medical Association* by a physician who had evaluated thirty-five different published studies on the use of drugs in the treatment of high blood pressure.[40] The author found to his surprise that every paper he'd looked at boasted either complete or significant partial relief from the material being tested. These papers variously claimed that mistletoe, diathermy, watermelon extract, even drops of dilute hydrochloric acid three times a day brought improvement in over 85 percent of the patients.

> Since all the substances tested were so radically different chemically one from the other, the author was forced to conclude that the only thing all the studies had in common was that 'the patients wanted to improve, they wanted their doctors to be successful, they wanted the drugs to work, they wanted to get better.' He attributed the successes in the studies to the well-known but little-discussed placebo effect.

Minding the Body

Glasser also reported an instance where two supposedly severely allergic patients could not be diagnosed. The patients were frustrated and angry that nothing could be found. All skin tests had been negative. A young doctor caring for them half-jokingly remarked that if only their skin tests would become positive, a diagnosis could be made, medications given and they would be cured. The next morning both patients had positive skin tests.

The mind controls the body in startling ways. People with so-called multiple personalities exhibit an interesting effect. Depending on which personality is present during the testing, they have been known to change physically in mind-boggling ways. A multiple may be allergic to some substance in one personality but not in another.

As well as doctors' explanations, media messages may provoke self-fulfilling prophecies. Consider the plight of those folks sensitive to the pollens that cause hay fever. Starting in August and lasting for months, the media report the pollen count. "The Pollen Count today is 5 (or 30 or 150)!" As it rises, we hear frequent predictions of how badly we are going to suffer. Sometimes we hear warnings to stay indoors.

The higher numbers are dis-easing seedthoughts. What good does it do to let people know these numbers? Since the amount of pollen in the air varies depending on where you are, on a low count day you might be near a high pollen area and react strongly. In this case, if you express yourself by hay fevering, you probably will have hay fever symptoms, whether you hear the pollen count or not. Constant warnings can harm those people who are highly susceptible to any hypnotic suggestion or particularly to pollen-related predictions.

In 1983 the media described the likelihood of a terrible year for hay fever sufferers. They reminded us that we'd had a wet spring and a hot, dry summer that encouraged more weeds and higher pollen levels. How many people who never had hay fever experienced symptoms that year? I met a few. The pollen count is meant to be helpful. But considering the creative power of beliefs, perhaps these warnings produce the opposite of their intended result. What can one do after hearing the pollen report—wear a mask?

Given the large numbers of messages of this nature that we receive every day, it is high time all of us learned to use positive affirmations and mental imaging techniques to counteract the negative messages that we hear and read. Pearsall writes about "a woman experiencing a severe hay fever reaction to pollen for twelve years. She was helped to imagine herself free of symptoms. She became completely free of her symptoms for the first time."[41]

Another distressing message was imparted by *People* magazine in its May 1989 issue. The cover story described the long-term effects of divorce on children of all ages. The statement on the cover was "Children of Divorce: Wounded Hearts." Think of the image that headline transmits: a memorable message to the subconscious mind. Frequent advertisements for this issue appeared on TV, so I bought a copy, to see how powerful the message was. I found this quote on the index page. "For years, psychologists thought that divorce was something kids got over, like chicken pox. But as those children know and a recent study has confirmed, the pain of a ruined marriage may linger in a child's life for years, causing confusion and heartache into adulthood."[42] The article itself, though it presented disturbing information, ended on a rather hopeful note, but these effects were subservient to the distressing headline.

You Get What You Believe

Two oft-quoted anecdotes regarding the effect of words on patients are provided by Bernard Lown, M.D., a professor of cardiology at Harvard University.[43] One woman heard her doctor say she was a classic case of T.S., which meant Tricuspid Stenosis or heart murmur—a common, non-serious condition. She was convinced TS meant "terminal situation." No amount of reassurance by others could reverse that belief and her doctor was nowhere to be located. She died later that same day despite determined efforts to save her.

A critically-ill heart attack patient was amazingly helped by a belief formed upon hearing his doctor's comment to the attending staff: "This patient has a wholesome, very loud third sound— gallop" (actually a poor sign that denotes that the heart muscle is straining and usually failing). The patient recovered. He said, "When I overheard you tell your colleagues I had a wholesome gallop, I figured I still had a lot of kick to my heart and could not be dying. My spirits were for the first time lifted, and I knew I would live and recover." Occasionally "ignorance is bliss." Sometimes "what you don't know won't hurt you." The words and thoughts of those around us can influence us positively or negatively. A workshop leader told me the following story:

> As a young boy, one of my clients had rheumatic fever. He was told repeatedly, 'Don't play—you may die.' Sometimes he played and felt faint, light-headed, or dizzy. These sensations supported the warning that he could die if he played too hard. In fact, the rheumatic condition this man had was a self-correcting type that is outgrown after adolescence. However, the now unconscious seedthought, 'Don't play or you'll die' had taken root in his mind-body system as a core belief.
>
> When he came to my workshop he had shut down to the joy and playfulness of life. During the workshop, he discovered the seedthought which was interfering with his aliveness and ability to participate fully in life. After the workshop he became much happier

and led a more productive life. You can counteract your harmful core beliefs just by being aware.

A woman named Faith gave me more evidence of the effect the words of adults have on children when she shared her story:

> When I was a little girl, I was severely bow-legged and walked pigeon-toed. My aunt told me, 'It hurts me to see that your leg isn't straight.' She then touched my leg and showed me how to straighten it and walk straighter.
>
> I loved this aunt deeply and was disturbed that she felt hurt. I thought about what she said quite often and attempted to keep my leg straight. But then, after a few days, the thoughts passed from my conscious mind and I just played and lived life normally. Several months later, my aunt noticed, and pointed out to me, that my leg was now straight. I was so thrilled to have pleased her. She didn't have to hurt for me anymore.

A man named Jim describes how he overcame the programming that limited him as a child:

> When I was growing up, I had difficulty walking, still falling often at five years of age. A doctor recognized the problem as Leg Perthes, a malformation of the hip joint. In the early 1940s this was not commonly diagnosed, nor were the doctors certain of the outcome of treatment. They prescribed no walking, bed rest, keeping pressure off the joint, and a full cast from my hips to my toes. Whether I would walk again was in doubt.
>
> I spent a year in bed, missing school till fourth grade. After the cast was removed, the last thing the doctors told my folks was, 'Encourage your son to study hard, so he can have a desk job. He will probably have difficulty with physical activity or exertion.' But my parents, especially my mother, bless her, always believed I would be perfect. So I believed it! She told me often, 'If you want something badly enough, you can have it.' She gave me faith in positive thinking.
>
> Today I am a soft drink distributor. My work is mostly physical: lifting, hauling, driving a truck. I play racquetball and exercise regularly. I believe that my mind can direct my body to do anything. I never take medicine, yet I haven't missed a day of work in 16 years. If I don't feel well, I rest and tell myself I will be well. Then I am

well! Every few years I have a physical checkup and the doctor says, 'You are perfect.'

Hope as Healer

Jim and Faith offer powerful testaments to the importance of being with people who believe in you and reassure you when you are feeling ill. Fear creates stress on the body. Prophets of doom upset the apple-cart of hope. Remember that hope isn't ever false, because a relaxed, trusting attitude creates a more favorable healing environment in the body. Don't ignore the reality of symptoms, check for organic causes, and expect a favorable outcome. Hope is a potent healing mechanism!

Even a developing fetus is affected by the thoughts and words of others. As we saw in earlier chapters, each emotion experienced in the mind produces its unique neuro-chemistry. These neurotransmitters produced in the brain of the pregnant woman then cross the placental barrier into the body of the developing baby. So when the pregnant woman feels shame, anger, or elation, the child's body chemistry changes to match.

The not-yet-born child responds to sounds as well as thoughts and feelings. During a TV show called "Cradle Hypnosis," psychologist John Bradshaw discussed these effects.[44] He cited the work of two Boston University researchers—Dr. William Condon and Dr. Louis Sander—who discovered that so-called random movements of infants immediately coordinated with speech. It seems that sounds heard prenatally program neuromuscular responses.

Using high-speed sound movies and computer analysis, Condon and Sander found that each infant had "a complete and individual repertoire of body movements which synchronized with speech." Every time a specific sound was made each infant responded with an individualized muscular response; whenever that sound was heard the response was always the same for that infant. Each child studied already had its own idiosyncratic responses to language. This programming began while the child was still in the mother's womb. It is thus conceivable that people's lives are affected by seedthoughts planted within them during their time in the womb. The words used in the presence of a pregnant woman can thus have far-reaching effects.

There is a biblical expression: "the truth will set you free." The truth is that *what we hear* affects *what we believe*. And what we believe affects whether we live or die, whether we are ill or well, whether we will prosper or wither on the vine.

Self-Help Experience #26
Helpful Reminders

Purpose: To practice presenting information in a more positive, useful, less accusatory way

Talk positively to others, using words, thoughts and images that suggest health, not disease. For example, it's better to say, "Eating vegetables and fruits will keep you healthier" rather than "If you don't eat right you'll get sick." The latter may be true but there is a positive way to present the information.

The mind remembers *the last few words* of a statement most vividly. How you phrase your warning statements is important. For example, it's better to say, "Remember to bring your homework" rather than "Don't forget your homework." The mind focuses on the last few words, in this case, "forget your homework."

For example:

Common	Better
Don't get sick.	Stay well.
Don't forget the milk.	Bring some milk home.
Cross streets carefully or you'll get hit.	Look both ways when crossing streets.
Be careful or you'll fall.	Hold on tight.
Study hard or you'll fail.	Study hard and you'll pass.
You're driving me crazy.	I get stirred up by you.
You'll be the death of me.	I worry about you.
You confuse me.	I don't understand you.

As you go through today, listen to your language for negative statements. Picture whatever image works for you: a watchdog or a gardener in your mind—sitting between your brain and your mouth—watching for and weeding out negative statements and changing them to positive ones. For example, labeling someone as stubborn rather than having a mind of his own.

Self-Help Experience #27
Feedback On Your Style

Purpose: To recognize the effect your way of speaking has on others

Instructions

1. Pay attention to the effect of your words on those around you. Choose a conversation with a friend to practice on today. First, practice being reassuring in everything you say.

2. Then switch to talking negatively.

3. Notice if your listener responds differently.

4. Finally tell the other person what you were doing. Ask them for feedback on how each mode of your talking affected them.

Self-Help Experience #28
Talking to Children

Purpose: To be more aware of the ways you talk to children, so you can choose your words more appropriately

Negative programming of young children is often glaringly apparent in waiting rooms at doctor's offices or in retail stores, especially supermarkets. I became aware of a shocking array of negative programming just listening to how parents talk to their children, especially when either parent or child is upset. For example: "Stop that or I'll kill you"; "You are driving me crazy"; "You'll never amount to anything."

Instructions

To encourage high self-esteem in children:

1. Start telling your child she *is already the way you want her to be.* For example, you might tell your baby, "You are a bright, cheerful baby." "You are handsome and friendly."

2. Pay attention to *good* behavior. When your child exhibits those ideals and behaviors which you value, reinforce them with praise. Don't emphasize the negative behaviors you observe. If you observe behavior you don't approve of, express your disapproval with an emphasis on the positive. Say something like, "Stop that! We prefer this...behavior instead."

3. Start now to use positive affirmations with your children, even if they are teenagers or older.

4. Believe your child can succeed in whatever she attempts. Don't berate her if she fails. Acknowledge her for trying.

5. Present your child with positive messages to enhance her self-confidence and self-esteem.

6. Encourage your child to practice making choices by offering her alternatives to choose from.

7.   Expect your child to have talents and she will. The talents might not be the ones you've hoped for. Respect the uniqueness and free choice of each individual.

The Operating Manual

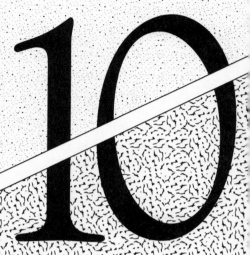

Scientists in a variety of interdisciplinary fields have concluded that there is one instrument in existence with the capability of advancing civilization beyond our present-day expectations. To date, this instrument has astounded owners by its broad range of innovative uses. Because it has tremendous value to society, there is a real desire to extend its life-span and enhance its daily operating ability. To maximize the potential of this instrument has become a primary concern of this decade.

Owners across the nation are faced with a common problem. This instrument does not come with Maintenance Instructions. Through years of ongoing experimentation, however, we have discovered that each owner must explore the available options and then create his or her own Operating Manual. Each owner is uniquely equipped to create this manual because each owner is the instrument referred to.

This instrument is, of course, the human being. We must learn how to care for this instrument if we are to maximize its potential and bring joy to its owners. Understanding mind/body communication is key. Being human is a wonderful gift!

The mind communicates with the body through language, thought, visual images, and metaphor. Seedthoughts program the body and emotions for either illness or wellness. The body talks back through physical sensations. The mind then gives these sensations meaning, providing information which stimulates more communication. This system operates continuously and automatically. A conscious mind can intervene and alter the system, for better or worse. Disease is part of the healing process.

Human bodies are composed of billions of cells which perform a vast array of electrical, mechanical and chemical functions. The body knows very well what it is doing. It functions by being in communication with each of its parts. Body machinery continuously operates without our conscious assistance. Organs and systems such as the digestive system communicate constantly without our supervision.

Consider your body as analogous to the hardware of the personal computer I write this book on. The body is the machine itself. However, something beyond the hardware (the body) is needed for the machine to operate: the software. To use my personal computer for writing I need word processing software that tells the computer what to do. As a human being you have some software built into your system, like the operating system of the computer. It's called the unconscious mind. You also have software that you generate by your thoughts, images, and words. Through your consciousness, you continuously program yourself throughout your life.

A properly programmed computer can perform functions unimaginable just fifty years ago. When programmed improperly, however, it will still malfunction. Similarly, an improperly programmed human mind causes the human system to malfunction. But properly programmed and maintained, *you* can perform beyond what was imaginable to most people fifty years ago. Witness the new inventions created to improve the quality of life, making it easier and faster to go, to get, to do almost anything. Witness also the feats of speed, stamina, endurance, and flexibility performed during the Olympic Games.

We are only beginning to test the limits of our achievements. By the end of the century, we may learn how to get along and trust others sufficiently to create enduring world peace. We may use our ingenuity to eradicate disease and eliminate starvation. We may travel at the speed of light. All this and more is possible for the healthy, well-maintained, finely developed human instrument. The key element in developing this potential is our level of consciousness.

Encouraging you to think for yourself and to create appropriate software is one of the aims of this book. But thinking for yourself also means aligning your thinking towards the Higher Self, the God Self that exists for and in all of us. Thinking derived from that Self leads to a desire for harmony and peace in the world. It leads to joining together in a common purpose for the good of all humankind.

Most computers have built-in feedback mechanisms which encourage internal correction before a total breakdown occurs. During a breakdown, the operator can make a correction if the malfunction is recognized in time. My personal computer is programmed with three options I can use to prevent some data disaster—abort, retry, or ignore. These options give me the chance to take action to avoid the disastrous loss of data.

A machine may beep or flash a red light to tell the operator that a correction is necessary. But the human body's red light is frequently a more subtle signal. It may be only vague discomfort, or intuition—that sixth sense—saying something is wrong. If the early warning signals are ignored, pain and disease often result. Disease is part of a human system's feedback.

Each part of the system gives feedback to the other parts. Your mind is the intelligence *operating* the system, and *observing* the system in operation. The system will operate more effectively and efficiently to the degree that you remain aware. Your body—the hardware—will be as good as the thoughts—the software—you program in, provided you keep ridding the system of outside interference as well as internal noise, distortions, and static.

Computers are subject to distortions due to static, or bugs in the system. The human system is also subject to distortions (dis-ease) due to static within—stresses caused by structural problems, poor diet, toxins, putrefied waste, germs, lack of rest, seedthoughts, and negative beliefs. Static distorts meaning in the human system, resulting in unclear communication from cell to cell, from organ to organ, and between mind and body. The human system continues to work, but static can lead to real damage in the body.

Distortion in the body affects the mind as well as vice versa. It's hard to think clearly when the body is in a weakened state. If toxins flow heavily in your blood stream, proper nourishment won't reach your brain. Poorly nourished brain cells can in turn result in unhealthy thoughts. Senility, for example, may be connected to brain cells dying from malnutrition. Most of the chronic, degenerative diseases appear to have some of these causal relationships. The immune system, the street patrol that keeps your body cleared of invaders, needs proper physical and mental nourishment to be in tip-top shape. If the distress in your system becomes too great, you shut down for a while and must go to bed while repairs are made. A computer crashes; you might need hospitalization.

Flying Blind

If I input an error into my computer, my data gets messed up. Once, while sampling a word processing program, I erased a whole disk by pressing keys whose function I didn't fully understand. Trying to operate a system without understanding the program is foolish—like flying blind. When I used the wrong input commands, I created the equivalent of disease in the computer and erased the disk. Trying to operate your body without understanding its design is also like flying blind. Many errors are based on insufficient information as to how to operate our human system. We often input unhealthy things, creating dis-ease.

Problems also exist because of the level of noise in our environment. Noise is analogous to the static in any machine or computer system. Noise is confused or confusing information. Noise is unhelpful, unwanted meaning! Noise in the human mind comes from your biases, belief systems, unhealthy seedthoughts, past experiences and memory. Noise distorts the messages you receive. To the extent that you are unaware of your biases, internal noise will color your perception of reality. Optimal health requires accurate information about what you feel and need. Distortion is the inability to perceive the true meaning of an event or sensation.

Intrapersonal Communication

When mind, body, and emotions are unified, each part of the system receives accurate communication. If a mind/body dichotomy prevails, error and distortion is more likely. If you are experiencing ill health, there may be a lack of clear and effective communication *from your body to your mind*. Ill health also signals that communication *from your mind to your body* probably contains unhealthy messages. This static in your intra-personal communication—you with yourself—can lead to illness.

In a recent article in *Smithsonian* titled "A Molecular Code Links Emotions, Mind And Health," Stephen S. Hall wrote, "The classic view of the body as three separate systems is challenged as research points the way to the new medicine of the 21st century....Some biologists believe we need to rethink some long-cherished principles, beginning with medicine's traditional separation of the central nervous system (the seat of thought, memory and emotion) from the endocrine system (which secretes powerful hormones) and the immune system (which defends the body from microbial invasions.)"[45]

Molecules carry messages amongst the various anatomical systems. These powerful biochemicals, called neurotransmitters or hormones, have been referred to as "informational substances" by M.I.T. neuroscientist Francis O. Schmitt. Some researchers say that learning how and why these substances work may influence medicine in the future similarly to the way genetic code research influenced medicine in the past. Further quoting Hall, "The informational substances, many of which are known to have a powerful effect on mood and emotion, provide a molecular way to understand the long-suspected connection between state of mind and state of health."[46]

Schmitt's biochemical information substances seem to be the vehicles that carry messages—thoughts and emotions—to cells throughout the body. These messengers then stimulate the production of other substances that enhance or detract from the body's functions. The mind, body, and emotions intersect in the immune system, which affects your ability to ward off disease. Anything in the nature of static in your system, whether physical or mental in origin, can produce unhelpful biochemical information. This pollution renders other systems less effective for the job they were meant to do.

Interpersonal Communication

Other people's words can contribute to the noise that prevents you from knowing what is true for you. A message from someone you love and trust can distort your own perception of reality. Static in interpersonal communication—you with others—can lead to unhappy personal relationships. If you aren't getting along with someone, there is probably some miscommunication or distortion of meaning. Distortion results in a breakdown in communication between individuals, families, and nations. Clear communication is always necessary for harmony.

Words often mean different things to different people. For example, take the word "upset." What do you mean when you say, "I am upset"? To some, "upset" means you are angry; to others, it means afraid; while to others, "upset" might indicate sadness. To complicate matters further, "I am upset" is a statement that means different things at different times. Now let's observe a sample dialogue to see how distorted communication can occur.

Mary says to John: "I feel really upset (meaning sad)."

John hears, "Oh, she's upset (meaning angry) with me. What did I do?"

John responds angrily: "What's wrong with you? What did I do to hurt you?"

Mary is flabbergasted. Why is John acting angry towards her when she is already so upset? Mary hasn't yet realized that John thinks she is angry at him.

Mary replies angrily: "I can't see why you're yelling at me when I feel this way."

John then goes on to justify his outburst and the two of them get further and further apart. These kinds of communication difficulties occur quite often, causing untold personal misery and damage to what might otherwise be good relationships.

Body Messages

Just as redundancy is built into this book for purposes of clarity, redundancy is part of the body's communication. Messages are repeated often, especially when they are ignored or misunderstood. Your body will speak louder and more clearly, until you get it.

For example, if I become accustomed to experiencing a dull ache in my lower back, I might come to accept it as inevitable. I may ignore it and not do anything about it. Thereafter, a dull ache in my lower back ceases to transmit any new information to me, information which might be useful for improving my state of health. Instead a louder message, perhaps intense sharp pain, would be necessary before I would take action. For me back pain leads me to my chiropractor. In years gone by, I needed lots of pain before I took that action. Now I am more aware of my body's structure.

Recently, my friend Anne, who has been quite overweight for many years, developed a kidney stone. After passing the stone she talked to me about about her weight. She said, "I've been waiting (weighting) for something to happen, some illness. I knew if I stayed fat something bad would happen to my body." Fear of suffering can be a potent motivating force. Anne's painful experience was her incentive to start exercising and change her diet.

Body weight messages are frequently ignored. Too much weight is often caused by eating too much of the wrong food. Also, eating too little of the right foods results in undernourishnment and the need for more food. The first message signaling poor eating habits might be feelings of tiredness, or an unsightly body. Our bodies usually signal us in the most benign ways possible. Ignoring the body's first weight message may result in more physical discomforts. The messages then get louder and clearer until they can no longer be ignored. High blood pressure, heart disease, liver and gall bladder troubles, and many more symptoms are related to improper eating habits.

Many years ago I had migraine headaches. For weeks at a time I would suffer bouts of intense pain. This was long before I knew anything about natural healing. I was mis-diagnosed as having "sinus headaches" and spent years on ineffective treatments. Later I received the accurate label of "cluster-migraine" but had no information as to the cause. Potent medicine eased the pain. Then I lost my voice so I quit smoking, thinking cigarettes were the cause of my laryngitis. Quitting had an unexpected benefit for me. I stopped having migraines. Years later I read that allergies to nicotine, alcohol, and other addictive substances can cause cluster-migraine headaches. The cause of my headaches had been obscured by my incomplete information. I wasn't sensitive enough to discern the harmful effects smoking was having on my body. Now my awareness of my body—my language connection—has strengthened significantly. My mind/body communication gets clearer all the time.

Highly sensitive medical technology is available to give you accurate biological feedback. This helps when you are unclear about the cause of a specific sensation or symptom. Most things that help you to know yourself better are very useful, and medical technology is no exception. Cardiograms, X rays, CAT scans, and the newer MRI scans, plus sophisticated chemical analysis of blood, hair, and urine can give you much-needed information. This diagnostic technology can catch potential breakdowns in your system before sickness makes you feel ill. Include in your Operating Manual these and other diagnostic techniques to be used when appropriate. Help your body to overcome the effects of noise in the system by periodic preventive maintenance in the form of checkups.

But the key to good health is static-free, accurate, intrapersonal communication: you with yourself and your mind with your body. Develop inner vision by uncovering your unconscious beliefs, just as peeling away the layers of an onion's skin releases its essence.

It is often useful to take a course which guides you towards this inner vision. Some are listed in the Appendix of this book. These are short-term training programs that came into vogue in the early seventies. The purpose of such courses is generally to help you to transform and improve the quality of your life. Participants usually report major breakthroughs in many areas of their lives.

Meditation classes or work with private counselors can also help you to de-stress, which always improves your internal communication. Increasing numbers of doctors are open to a variety of healing modalities and will often assist you in finding the way. Static-free self-communication is available to anyone willing to invest time and energy in the process.

Sometimes it's useful to go on retreat and immerse yourself in an intensive program to get to know yourself better. The Kripalu Center for Yoga and Health in Massachusetts is one such place. Kripalu offers many programs designed to improve your well-being. One three-week program called "Kripalu Health for Life" combines many of the elements that promote good health: good diet; exercise; bodywork; relaxation training; plus hours of experiential workshops, many of which enhance self-awareness. The program includes a comprehensive medical assessment and ongoing medical support.

Kripalu reports the following documented results:

- Hypertension—80% of those using medication prior to the program significantly reduced or eliminated their need for medication;

- Cholesterol—those with above normal levels achieved an average 15% decrease;

- Triglycerides—average drop 15%;

- Diabetes—all participants with adult-onset diabetes decreased or eliminated their need for medication;

- Weight—average loss 8 pounds for those desiring to lose weight.[47]

The Truth Process

The "truth process" is an important technique to include in your Operating Manual. When you can objectively observe yourself and then truthfully describe to yourself what you are feeling, you will know yourself better. I first recognized this during my est training in 1973. *est* is an acronym for Erhard Seminars Training. But est also means "it is" in French and Latin, so est is about finding the truth about the way "it" (life) is for you at any given moment in time. During the "truth process," a guided exercise, we practiced telling the truth about what we were experiencing, instead of fooling ourselves with excuses and illusions. An objective witness doesn't get sucked in by the lies of the mind.

If I have a headache, I stop what I am doing and observe it ("experience it" was the est term). I stay emotionally detached and describe the shape, color, and temperature of the sensations I feel in my head. It helps to have someone ask me questions about those qualities. Some people feel silly doing this, but it is a very effective technique, especially with children. I then observe any meaning I attach to the physical sensations I label "headache," looking for reasons to explain what I am experiencing.

I scan my memory banks for all the causes I have ever associated with headache, such as allergy, not enough sleep, or too much sun. Discovering the cause can help prevent future headaches. Now that I no longer smoke and I eat more carefully, I am relatively headache-free. When I do have a headache, my body has sent an effective warning signal, communicated to me through pain, that some change is in order. I get the message!

During the est training, each trainee selected a problem to focus on. While thinking about the condition which we hoped to eliminate—perhaps a headache or an emotion such as jealousy—we described to ourselves the physical sensations and emotions that we were feeling. We noted the thoughts we were thinking. Doing this process taught me to objectively witness myself.

Afterwards, many trainees talked about the releases that they achieved during the truth process. It seems that by minutely observing and describing their experience at that moment, they caused the sensations, emotions, and the experience itself to vanish. I am not sure why observing a painful condition makes it disappear. The explanation given us by the trainer was "When you fully experience your experience it will disappear." To me that meant that *we are supposed to learn something from each of our experiences, and when we do, we can move on to the next experience.* By objectively observing ourselves we extract the necessary information to learn from whatever happens in our lives.

Ultimately the self-attention of witnessing will expand your understanding of each event in your life and the effects of these events on you. Understanding leads to increased awareness of how you need to act to care for your human instrument to achieve a better quality of life.

Self-Help Experience #29
Creating Your Own Self-Help Manual

Purpose: To build your own self-help resource. Get a loose leaf notebook and divide it into sections with headings such as:

Exercise Instructions. Include exercises from this book or from other sources that you've found helpful.

Results of Different Experiences. Use this section to record what you observed, thought, and felt as you used the self-help experiences at the end of each chapter.

Daily Diary. Use the diary section to record the events of your day. Take a minute or two each day to at least jot down the highlights of your day. The greater the detail, the more you will learn about yourself. Include your evaluation of any event. For example: lunch with John—Fun, but I felt exhausted from so much talking. Roller skating with Phil—He's easy to be with. Nautilus workout—Great. Fight with boss—What a drag.

Tristine Rainer in *The New Diary* recommends using a diary to understand the meaning of an illness. Write a dialogue with the specific part of the body or the specific illness that is giving you trouble. One woman discovered that her bronchitis was the voice of her previously unexpressed anger. She promised herself to speak up and the bronchitis promised to go away.[48]

Decisions. List pros and cons to help you decide.

Goals. Write what you hope to achieve—today, in a week, a month, a year, five years, and so on.

Miscellaneous. Since this is your Operating Manual, you will choose the appropriate sections to include. My mom had a book she called her bible. In it was important material related to her life, such as medical and financial information, appointment data, favorite activities, etc.

Self-Help Experience #30
Understanding Pain Messages

Purpose: To improve your general level of health. The body is as logical as a computer; *what you program in is what you get*. The design function of pain is to make you aware of a malfunction which has the potential of making your system inoperative. When you first experience a pain, you need to stop and ask yourself some questions.

Instructions

1. *What does the pain mean?* The answer to this question will lead you to the appropriate treatment. Don't panic. Clear decoding of body signals is essen-

tial. For example, if you experience chest pain, there are many possible explanations. Check the meaning of the message by noticing any *accompanying body messages*. Are you nauseous? sweating? short of breath? Does the pain radiate? Does your heart palpitate? If you have these symptoms and are over a certain age, you might label your pain as heart attack.

If accompanying your pain in the chest you are having chills, fever, symptoms of cold and flu, you might suspect pneumonia. Chest pains can be caused by a broken rib, by a burst air sac in the lung, indigestion, gallstones, pulled muscles, or other factors.

2. *What have I been doing to/or with my body?* Your body tells you through sensation if you are acting inappropriately. If your hand starts to feel too hot, you're too close to the fire. Are you eating right, too much, too little, healthy foods? Exercising enough, or too much? Are you spending quiet time with yourself? What kinds of thoughts have been dwelling in your mind?

3. *What actions do I need to take to relieve these symptoms and improve my body?* Sit quietly for a few minutes and reflect on your answers to the above questions. Then the answer to this question will flow from the information you've received. You will know what to do or who to see to guide you into appropriate treatment.

4. *Take action.* Use the pain message to improve the quality of your life by acting on what you've learned. For example: I discovered some food allergies were causing me to itch so I stopped eating those foods. If you think you have pneumonia, see a doctor, and follow his instructions. If you have frequent headaches and recognize a cause, eliminate that cause from your life. Act on what you learn from any discomfort you experience. Get the message!

Self-Help Experience #31
The Truth Process

Purpose: To discover truth and relieve pain. To release unwanted behavior patterns such as jealousy, insecurity or procrastination.

Sue, the woman we met in an earlier chapter recognized her seedthought, "I don't want to hear that," during the truth process and freed herself of recurrent ear infections. This non-judgmental witnessing can be used to ease any pain, whether physical or emotional in origin.

With physical pain, first do exercise #30 to understand any pain messages. You might be resisting the pain by tensing your body, thus making matters worse. Your physical sensations will probably change during this process before the pain leaves completely. Your focused attention can cause the pain to intensify momentarily, but it will usually ease quickly.

Instructions

1. When you are experiencing pain, stop what you are doing and observe it. Don't ignore it. Experience it completely. If you are using this process to release an emotion or change an unwanted behavior pattern, begin by thinking about the behavior.

2. Notice your state of mind and emotions related to the sensations you are feeling and the thoughts you are thinking. Are you angry, sad, frustrated, etc.?

3. Stay emotionally detached as you *describe the shape, color, and temperature* of any sensations you feel. It helps to have someone ask you questions about those qualities. Pretend your pain or emotion has a color and a shape.

4. What meaning do you attach to your physical sensations? Scan your memory banks for past causes of similar sensations. What reasons explain or justify your pain?

5. Is there any situation in your present life that might be contributing to this current pain or upset?

6. Recall any earlier, similar situations related to the one you are now experiencing.

7. Go through these steps 1–6 a second time.

8. Thank your body and your mind for what the discomfort is teaching you.

9. Acknowledge any new truth you have learned. Write it in your Operating Manual or journal.

Self-Help Experience #32
Relaxation Activities

Purpose: To center yourself and clear mental distractions during an upset. Read through the following list of possibilities. Some may seem odd and not in keeping with your temperament. Some you will be drawn to try. Set time aside for some relaxation activities each day. Be open to new activities and new hobbies.

Instructions

1. Walk barefoot on the beach or grass. This works even in cold weather.

2. Hug a tree. It may sound silly but try it anyway. Trees really are our friends, and their continuity of being is a valuable reminder of the central values at the core of life.

3. Read something you normally don't read.

4. Become a couch potato and vegetate for a time. Teenagers call it "vegging out."

5. Fly a kite.

6. Read the Bible.

7. Listen to a guided meditation tape.

8. Play spiritual music. Anything from hymns to New Age music can induce relaxation.

9. Get up and dance to your favorite music.

10. Do some art work or any creative activity.

11. Do anything "just for the fun of it."

12. List your favorites in your Operating Manual.

When the going gets tough, the tough get going
Count your blessings
A stitch in time saves nine

Keys to the Good Health Kingdom

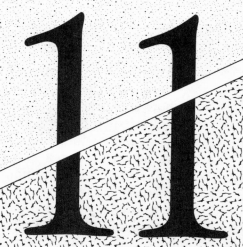

We each have an ongoing inner dialogue. A voice of judgment speaks to us continuously, analyzing and evaluating our experience. ("What voice?" you may ask. "The one that asked that question!" I would answer.) Through introspection, a kind of meditation on oneself, one is able to process the pleth- ora of signals one has to deal with each day, to make sense out of the complex stimuli in our internal and external environment.

Life works according to your ability to process information clearly, effectively, and meaningfully. A healthy, purposeful existence and rewarding relationships with others requires practice in coding and decoding, as well as time for the prac- tice to be effective. Through years of training, I have become expert at witnessing myself in a relatively objective way, and clearly describing what I experience, usually (but not always) without judging or condemning myself. It was this ability to witness myself that enabled me to write this book from a point of personal understanding. Witnessing myself and com- ing to grips with my own experience taught me empathy for others.

Intuition

Intuition, the direct knowledge or awareness of something without conscious attention or reasoning, will tell you when to see a doctor, when to get some exercise, when to rest. We all have some degree of intuition whether we pay attention to it or not. I know when I need a chiropractic adjustment, even if I can't describe any strong sensations. I feel something, and I have learned to interpret and trust what I feel. Perhaps people with reliable intuition know how to keep the static out of their feedback system. Perhaps intuitive people have a strong language connection, fine-tuned by their ability to decode body messages.

My daughter Jennifer has a well-developed intuitive sense. She often says, "I don't know why, but something tells me I should do this," or "A voice inside me tells me not to eat this." When she was younger she said the voice was separate from her (and maybe it was). But now she says it's a part of herself that she trusts. Intuitively you can know what ails you long before it can be medically verified. A patient of Westport psychiatrist Harry Brown had a dream about wanting to eat red meat and blood. Dr. Brown said, "She was distressed by her dream. I recommended she take a blood test, and we found she was anemic." She tapped her inner knowledge and dreamt a signal for her mind to act on. She was then guided by a skilled physician who became her partner in taking corrective action.

The mind/body/emotions represent a continuous, closed-circuit communication system with instantaneous feedback. Meditation provides a pathway to clearer self-communication, a way to reconnect the seemingly separate parts of your system and bring back health. Developing your intuition is a side benefit. Meditation involves experiencing a quieter mind, without the judgmental thoughts and memories that often intrude on your experience. During meditation you more easily recognize the messages coming from your body, your emotions, and your subconscious mind. You can eliminate the noisy interference of unproductive, unhealthy thoughts—freeing yourself from the distortions that cause disease.

Varieties of Meditation

In some meditation systems you are told to sit with a straight spine or lie flat on your back with eyes closed. Observe your breath by focusing your attention on inhaling and exhaling. If you start thinking about something else, your attention has wandered from your breath. Don't think about the thoughts, just notice them, and return your awareness to your breath. Some teachers tell you to follow the path of your breath as it travels through your body. For me, that means to imagine where the air I breathe goes after entering my body.

Another meditation system involves the repetition of a mantra. A mantra is a word or syllable with spiritual significance and special creative power. A mantra can either be repeated inwardly or chanted out loud. The focus on the word or phrase keeps the mind occupied. Most religions have some form of this meditation: the Christian "Hail Mary," the Hebrew "Sh'ma Yisrael," Hindu "Om Nama Shivaya," the Buddhist "Nam Myoho Renge Kyo," or the sacred sound "Aum" or "Om" used in many systems.

Different teachers train or initiate people in the use of their favored tones, sounds, and words. One system I like includes chanting the vowels of the English alphabet and imagining a specific color with each vowel sound. Some people achieve good results just counting "one, two," bringing on the relaxation necessary for meditation.

In the Judeo-Christian tradition, meditation is often called contemplation. Meditation may either make you more present and more aware (to know your self better), or conversely, less present and less aware (to forget yourself and know God better). Each state is beneficial.

Quieting the mind by focusing one-pointedly on one thing, be it your breath, a specific prayer, or a mantra, takes practice. Daily sessions of at least twenty minutes are recommended, preferably before a meal. Steady use of these relaxing techniques eventually filters out the thoughts that prevent you from hearing and understanding your inner self.

Many claims have been made regarding the effectiveness of meditation. Long-time meditators often report that they feel more relaxed; need less sleep; think more clearly; and cope better with stress, among other claims. Many people who have experienced remission of a chronic or terminal disease note that meditation, in one form or another, was a key part of their healing program.

Researchers at the Medical Center of the University of California at Irvine found that the practice of Transcendental Meditation increased the flow of blood to the brain. "The average increase in blood flow in participants was 65% greater than that measured when the subject merely relaxed. This may account, at least in part, for the role of meditation in improved mental performance observed in earlier studies."[49]

Alcoholics use drink to cope with stress. A *Brain/Mind Bulletin* article reports that practicing meditation gives alcoholics another coping tool. Two Chicago doctors—alcoholism program treatment directors—emphasize that "these procedures must not be thought of as a form of treatment but as an adjunct to medical and psychiatric approaches during the period of acute withdrawal."

Brain/Mind Bulletin also reports on the helpfulness of meditation in reducing alcoholic drinking in general, in heavy social drinkers. In one study of different relaxation therapies to support reduced drinking, meditation (Benson's relaxation response) was found to be the "best option for alcoholism treatment among several treatments evaluated."[50] Other options were progressive muscular relaxation and "bibliotherapy," restful reading twice daily. A control group received no therapy at all. It seems that subjects taught to meditate were most likely to continue the relaxation program and thus achieved more lasting reduction in their alcohol consumption.

A study of the effects of Transcendental Meditation on prisoners incarcerated in Folsom prison in California indicated significant enhancement in mental health. A three-month study of 26 prisoners and 30 controls examined anxiety, neuroticism, hostility, aggressive behavior, self-concept, resting blood pressure, and pulse rates. Pre-test and post-test smoking and sleep patterns also were studied for the meditating prisoners. After three months, the TM subjects were "less anxious, less prone to violence, more stable and had an improved self-concept." After the study was completed, there was a waiting list of 500 prisoners wanting to be trained in the technique.[51]

Meditation can help many conditions. Henry Reed, Virginia Beach psychologist and dream research authority, conducted a study with members of A.R.E.—The Association for Research and Enlightenment. It was discovered that meditation improves dream recall, at least in experienced meditators.[52] The New York telephone company adopted meditation as part of its regular health maintenance program after an eighteen-month study on stress reduction involving 154 employees.[53] Other experiments using meditation have demonstrated its value in reducing hypertension.[54]

Mindfulness

The Zen concept of meditation is mindfulness, in which you stay aware of your present reality without the distraction of extraneous thoughts. For example, when you are washing the dishes, you keep all your attention on washing the dishes, so that you fully experience washing the dishes. Since it's not possible to focus clearly on two thoughts at one time, worry tends to disappear during mindfulness. Stated simply, it means doing whatever you do with an attitude of total absorption.

Witnessing yourself is a form of mindfulness in which you focus inwardly on all you are experiencing at any given moment, including your thoughts and feelings. The witness, an objective observer, is *you watching you* without judgment. The idea is to detach yourself from your surroundings so that all attention is focused on your inner process.

I often find this difficult. My mind wants to wander, think of other things, do its own activity. It takes effort and strong intention to control my mind. Recently during a meditation, I encountered a potent visual metaphor for the objective observer observing myself. Each time, a large blue eye appeared in my visual field, though my eyes were closed. The eye (I) was watching me. The blue eye was the "I" of my Self, watching me even while I watched It. If your mind continually dwells on a problem, writing it out in your journal is useful, as it saves the data without your constantly needing to re-play the mental tape.

The descriptions of mindfulness, insight, and witnessing are based on my own experience of the meaning of these terms and may not be the same as the meaning used by any specific group. When the mind is quieted by any means, you gain insight—that special sense of "seeing things as they really are." Your expanding awareness leads to more appropriate lifestyle choices.

All systems of meditation take practice, self-discipline, and an attitude of calm, centered acceptance of oneself. The rewards of each form of.meditation are great, proportionate to the disciplined effort of the meditator, just like any other self-improvement activity. To meditate is to put into practice the desire to be increasingly in touch with your inner world. Meditation can be practiced in a variety of ways throughout the day.

Moving Meditations

Not all meditation practices are done sitting quietly. There are also moving meditations. Examples include Tai Chi, Hatha Yoga, and many of the martial arts. Of course, the movement alone is beneficial to the body. But in each of these systems, the mental focus on the activity results in a release of tension in mind and body.

My favorite activity for relaxation, meditation, and exercise is walking. During walking I solve problems, gain inspiration for writing, use affirmations, exercise my body, and reduce stress by releasing negative energy. I am in charge of my mind's activity during a walk. But if I am agitated about some real or imagined problem, my mind often takes charge and runs through its memory bank of tapes related to my problem. I allow this process to go on for a while because I learn about my unconscious feelings by observing my upsetting thoughts. I can then improve my situation.

Dancing is effective as social activity, for gaining fitness, destressing,and releasing emotion. Classical ballet, jazz, folk, and social dancing often require focused attention to perform them properly. Music helps us reach the non-conscious mind. Just listening to music often unlocks the door that seems to block feelings and thoughts, allowing images to arise spontaneously. Images are the door to the not-yet-conscious, and music is the key which unlocks it. Any physical activity where you are fully involved—with music or without—can become a kind of meditation.

Personal Prayer

Personal prayer is another form of meditation which absorbs the mind. It can be practiced sitting in stillness or moving around. You may use your own words or something like the Lord's Prayer or Biblical verses. The Gayatri Mantra and the World Invocation are other ways to use a prayer-focused mind to achieve a specific result in the world. The Bible says: "Therefore I tell you, whatever you ask for in prayer, believe that you have received it, and it will be yours." (Mark 11:24, New International Version) A favorite prayer of mine is the Serenity Prayer: "God grant me the serenity to accept the things I cannot change, the will and courage to change the things I can, and the wisdom to know the difference."

Prayer is effective whether you pray for yourself or if others pray for you. In the recent case of the jogger brutally attacked in Central Park, thousands, maybe millions of people prayed for her. Her recovery thus far has been way beyond the expectations of her doctors. In another case, the whole world waited for Jessica McClure to be rescued from the well in Texas. Then too, our prayers were answered.

A double blind randomized study by cardiologist Randy Byrd using 393 coronary care unit patients at San Francisco General Hospital adds weight to the belief that patients have fewer medical complications when prayed for. 192 patients were prayed for and 201 were not. Neither patients nor Dr. Byrd were aware of who was being prayed for until the data was recorded. The people praying were told the patients' first names and diagnoses. Byrd had recruited Christians and Jews from all over to pray for several patients each, in whatever form they chose. Statistics showed the two groups of patients were equally sick when they entered the hospital, but that patients who were prayed for had fewer complications during their stay.[55]

During meditation or prayer, as you unify your mind/body/emotions and reconnect your seemingly separate parts, you expand your ability to choose freely. You ensure yourself of clearer mind/body communication. You will know yourself better. You will begin to recognize and accept your emotions, uncover harmful beliefs and seedthoughts, and begin to change them through the power of creative thinking. Joyfully accept it! An attitude of gratitude is a primary ingredient for a happy, healthy, peaceful, fulfilled life.

Self-Help Experience #33
Mindfulness Meditation

Purpose: To practice witnessing yourself without judgment

Instructions

Practice each one of the four categories below by itself for a few sessions of ten minutes each, until you gain proficiency in the technique. Sit straight with eyes closed. Later, after combining all the categories to practice the complete meditation, you will be able to effectively witness yourself throughout the day, even with your eyes open.

1. *Sensations from inside your physical body.* Focus attention on your physical body, watching your breath rise and fall. Note posture, physical attributes, and body sensations such as:

    Taste
    Temperature
    Muscular tension
    Color or lack of color behind your eyelids
    Hunger pangs
    Pain

    Note whether the sensation is pleasant, unpleasant, or neutral. Because the mind works by classifying, you observe your mind classifying. You may realize that thoughts have a creative life of their own.

2. *Sensations from outside your body.* Note sensations arising external to your body, such as:

    The feel of air moving across your body.
    The touch of the object you are sitting on.
    The air temperature where you are sitting.
    The kinds of sounds you hear. Is it quiet, noisy, calming, distracting?
    Is your sitting space brightly lit or darkened?
    Does the space feel cramped or roomy?
    Note whether the sensation associated with each item is pleasant, unpleasant, or neutral.

3. *Your state of mind.* Note your state of mind and how it shifts. Are you annoyed, impatient, at peace? Each time a new state appears, note "mind impatient," "mind peaceful," "mind doubting," or even "mind eager."

4. *Visual pictures and memories.* Note any visual pictures or memories that come to mind. Notice how you classify thoughts and evaluate them. There will be some overlapping of categories when you begin to practice, but that is fine because ultimately you will incorporate all the categories into a combined practice.

5. *Combined Practice.* After practicing each of the four categories singly for several sitting sessions, you will be ready for combined practice. Plan to sit about 40 minutes. Your basic focus is on the breath. As you sit, observing your breath and posture, be ready to receive other impressions. Whatever you experience is to be noted, be it sensation, thought, feeling, or state of mind. When you have no other thoughts or experiences, when no other mindfulness category is operating, return to observing your breath.

Eventually mindfulness will become your usual state. This monitoring may be difficult, even uncomfortable, but the results are remarkable, according to Justin Stone, from whose book *Meditation For Healing* this exercise is adapted. "For the first time we see how we actually operate; for the first time we have self-knowledge."[56] The mental delusions we subject ourselves to can disappear, healing sickness in the mind.

Self-Help Experience #34
A Ten-Step Plan to Improve Your Life

Purpose: A daily routine that will improve the quality of your life. Gandhi is reported to have said, "Total effort, total victory."

Instructions

1. Keep a journal of your feelings every day.
2. Join a support group that meets at least once a month. Every week is better if you are in crisis or ill.
3. Live an hour at a time.
4. Meditate, pray, or listen to music at least once or twice a day.
5. Do some form of physical exercise each day.
6. Eat what you believe is a good diet.
7. While looking in the mirror, repeat aloud, "I love you (add your name)." Occasionally do this in front of a mirror while naked. Notice any negative judgments you have about yourself and cancel them.
8. Give thanks to a higher power for the good in your life. Give thanks, too, for the trials you face. Learn something from them.
9. Hug at least one person every day.
10. Tell at least one person every day that you love them.

Self-Help Experience #35
Personal Prayers

Purpose: To connect you with a higher power

If you think you don't know how to pray, relax! It's just like talking to someone you love and trust, in your own words, in silence or aloud, wherever you happen to be—sitting, standing, walking, lying down, or even driving. Prayer is real and potent and comes from your heart when you choose the words. This is my favorite daily prayer for guidance and protection:

"Mother-Father-God, just now I ask for your presence, through the light of the Christ and the Holy Spirit. Please fill, surround, and protect me with your radiant light. I give thanks for all that I have received. (Sometimes I give thanks for specific things.) I ask that only that which is for my highest good and the highest good of all will occur. Thank you! I ask that the light and the Holy Spirit be sent to (names of family members, friends, business associates, and world situations)."

Self-Help Experience #36
Who's Responsible for Me?

Purpose: To accept personal responsibility for your life without condemning or judging yourself

Remind yourself daily until the idea becomes second nature, "I am responsible for my life. I choose what to think and feel. Responsibility does not imply blame, shame, or a negative evaluation of myself. Responsibility is merely my acceptance (without judgment) of the control I do have over my life."

Expect the best; be prepared for the worst
Every day, in every way,
I am getting better and better

Healing Techniques:
Self-Hypnosis, Visualization, Affirmation & Chanting

12

In a guided meditation you follow a series of instructions during which you actively use your creative imagination. Guided meditations are useful when you know what is needed in order to heal yourself because you can imagine that effect. For example, you might imagine: more antibodies to release a virus; a tumor getting smaller each day; you becoming slimmer; you swimming rather than smoking; etc. The use of mental imagery rests on the basic assumption that through our minds we can affect our bodies. Simply demonstrated, this is the principle behind thinking about tasting sweet chocolate and discovering that you salivate as a result of the thought, just as if the real chocolate had been thrust into your mouth.

Picturing What You Want

Visualization is often part of a guided meditation. After quieting the mind using any of several techniques, the now relaxed meditator imagines a specific result. Some are good at visualizing and see clear images. Others sense or feel the desired change in different parts of the body. Some hear or think words to guide the creative force within them. It's

145

possible to achieve most goals with visualization. Corporate planners relate the value of visualization to ideas like management by objective, targeting and goal setting.

Since visualization can be used to produce almost any desired result, it's a great aid in achieving your goals. Brian Boitano, upon winning the 1988 Olympic Gold Medal for figure skating said, "It was my dream performance that I'd visualized a million times, at least once a day, since I was nine years old."

Mental imagery for medical purposes has been used increasingly throughout the 1980's. Kenneth Pope of the Brentwood, California Veterans Adminsitration hospital, speaking at the first annual conference devoted to mental imagery said, "mental imagery of blood vessels increasing in diameter, in combination with general relaxation, helps hypertensive patients lower their blood pressure. Those using relaxation alone were less effective." He went on to explain that verbal language was limited in its effect on the autonomic nervous system. Telling your blood pressure to drop just doesn't do it. On the other hand, "the autonomic nervous system responds to a more basic language—imagery."[57]

Psychoanalyst Gerald Epstein believes that "People have to see that the mind, using imagery, can repair the body." He reports the case of a man with chronic eczema, who was given an exercise to do three times a day for three weeks. Detailed instructions included "imagining his fingers becoming palm leaves which he put on his face." To finish the exercise he was to see his face becoming all clear. First the eczema moved from his face to his body and then cleared completely.[58]

A woman with arthritis was given an imaging exercise that shrunk by 3 1/2 inches an eight-inch rheumatoid nodule in her right knee. A man facing prostate surgery had a normal prostate after doing a simple imagery twice daily for six months.[59]

Using mental imagery may even enhance visual perception. According to research psychologist Ronald Finke, you might see something more quickly if you first imagine it. "Suppose you are flying an airplane through a cloud, you might see the runway sooner if you were to imagine it in advance at its proper location. If on the other hand, you imagined it at a different location, you might take longer to see it correctly than if you had not imagined it at all."[60] You see what you believe and if you don't believe it, you probably won't see it.

Polar Bears Can Chill Cancer

Erik Esselstyn is a living example of the effectiveness of visualization and facing emotions in the long-term cure of cancer. He tells the following story:

> In 1976, I developed bile duct cancer, a rare form of cancer, difficult to diagnose and treat. Extensive surgery removed the cancer and parts of my stomach, pancreas, duodenum, gall bladder and common bile duct.
>
> The prognosis after this surgery was poor so, after reading about visualization as a weapon against cancer in the Simonton's book *Getting Well Again,* I began to do visualization twice a day for twenty minutes. First I would use a mantra-based meditation to relax and to release static energy from my system. Then I would visualize an army of white polar bears I recruited to assist me in my cancer battle. I saw countless imaginary polar bears coursing through my bloodstream and lymphatic system, always on the lookout for cancer cells, always ready to devour them.
>
> I chose the polar bears because they are brave, resolute hunters, and persistent survivors. Their white color clearly relates to the body's white blood cells. Trooping through my system they searched out and devoured any lingering cancer cells. Other images could work, but the white polar bear, warm and fuzzy in my mind, remains a lifelong friend and ally searching out the dark, "grapefruit-sized" cancer cells.
>
> For two years after the surgery I would feel/sense the polar bears zapping the ugly cancer cells. I knew each time another cancer cell was gone. At the end of each visualization session, the victorious polar bears met at the top of my brain, with thumbs up for victory.
>
> I have continued this procedure since leaving the hospital in 1976. After two years I stopped feeling the sensation I called, 'a cancer cell being zapped.' My polar bears no longer encounter any of the grapefruit-sized menaces. While I believe all traces of the disease are gone, I still continue the visualization twice daily, sending my polar bear army on its mission through my system as a precaution against disease. The malignancy has never recurred. I am deeply

grateful to the surgeon who performed the lifesaving surgery and to the Simontons for their self-help techniques.

Another patient visualized white knights on horseback running through her body, doing battle with the black cancer cells. The white knights symbolized antibodies at work. Another was a pacifist who refused to kill her cancer. She visualized herself carrying the malignant cells out of her body.

Besides eliminating errant cancer cells, visualization can help destroy bacteria and viruses, reduce tumors, heal broken bones and restore organic function in any part of your body. Visualization is also a preventive technique, stimulating immunity when used before overt signs of cancer or other disease. One can see the problem shrinking, burning up, erased, dissolved, or washed out of the body. Visualization has even been reported to help well-trained individuals in prevention or encouragement of conception.

Affirmations

Dr. Emmett Miller, M.D., Medical Director of the Cancer Support and Education Center in Menlo Park, California, and author of the book *Self-Imagery,* specializes in psycho-physiological medicine and stress reduction. He created *Software for the mind,* a series of audio cassette tapes that provide the brain with clear, easy-to-comprehend "programs" designed to support self-healing, stress reduction, personal change and optimal performance.

One patient used the surgery tapes before and after a radical hysterectomy and partial lymphectomy. She said, "The tape prepared me completely for what to expect, step-by-step; the shock and surprise were eliminated. The tape took me deep into my body and left me with a sense of well- being." Her surgeon called her recovery remarkable. Another used the surgery tapes before having a cancerous lung removed, a difficult operation for both surgeon and patient. Her doctor said that her recovery was the fastest he'd seen from this type of surgery.

Affirmations are consciously chosen seedthoughts one inserts in the subconscious mind in order to produce a certain result. Dr. Miller says,

To change mental programming and create new, health-producing software, a key element is repetition. The unhealthy thought patterns were usually created over time, by your repeatedly thinking the same thoughts. To improve health, performance, and creativity you must think just as repeatedly in the newer way.

Some of our requests to our brains are immediately followed by the appropriate behavior. Yet requests or demands to stop smoking, eat less, have a positive attitude, overcome a phobia of snakes, or stop feeling pain are seldom acted upon. This is because these behaviors—though felt consciously to be wrong—are stored unconsciously in the mind. When these same requests are offered as positive suggestions, images, and affirmations, they are more easily accepted, especially when the person has been guided into a relaxed, receptive state. In this state one is exquisitely receptive to new 'programs' which are offered in 'brain language'—positive affirmations, autosuggestions, and experience-based, sensory-rich imagery. We can improve our lives by making positive changes in our software.

One man had his leg amputated below the knee. He had such great difficulty using an artificial leg that he couldn't walk. His skin kept ulcerating, causing a great deal of pain. During a hypnotherapy session he re-created the incident where his leg was lost, recalling his last thought as the leg was being blown off: "Now I'll never walk again." Using Miller's guided imagery tape he recreated the accident and imagined a different thought. He told himself repeatedly, "My leg is gone but I shall walk again using an artificial leg." He repeated this affirmation and saw himself walking. Within a few days, the skin on his leg healed, he was freed from pain and he was able to wear the prosthesis.

Another patient used relaxation tapes to cure a hair-trigger temper. While in the relaxed state, he practiced dealing with difficult situations without anger. He rehearsed by first imagining provocative situations and then his calm reactions—many times over. At the end of each day, he reviewed every challenge to his calmness, praising his successes and visualizing a better way if he had handled the situation poorly. After a week, he reported major improvement in this behavior pattern.

Hypnosis

According to hypnotherapist Linda Zelizer:

> Hypnosis is powerful, safe and easy to use. During hypnosis you are in an altered state, during which your critical conscious mind is less active and more open to changes. Hypnosis has helped many people to stop smoking, lose weight, overcome fears and phobias, reduce pain, eliminate insomnia, heal physical conditions, and improve both memory and concentration.
>
> Hypnosis works with your inner mind which influences every-thing you do. The power of hypnosis is in the mind's receptivity to suggestions during the altered state of awareness. You can then move past your *learned limitations* and focus your energy on new ways of thinking and behaving. You are never out of control so you won't say or do anything which goes against you. Hypnosis won't even make you do something you think you should do, but don't really want to do—like stop smoking.
>
> One technique, Hypnotic Exploration, used with a professional hypnotherapist, can help you to find the irrational thinking that is linked to the behavior you desire to change. Then in the hypnotically altered state, your chosen suggestions can help you to reprogram your beliefs and attitudes. Changing is then easier, more effective and more permanent. With such a potent resource, there's no longer a reason to believe that change is impossible.

Prenatal memories and birth trauma affect individuals well into adulthood according, to a growing body of research evidence. Hypnosis can help unlock the hidden memories so healing can take place. "Many people have recalled pre-natal and birth experiences that related to current physical and psychological problems: headaches, respiratory disorders, phobias, depression, anxiety. Recalling the experiences frequently relieves or eliminates the symptoms."

A male client of therapist Jack Downing relived a painful fetal memory of rejection while under hypnosis. This was verified when his mother said that his father had indeed wanted her to have an abortion upon learning of the pregnancy. Gynecologist David Cheek says his patients' ability to recall details of their birth is uncanny. He checks details, verifying their accuracy using obstetrical notes made during delivery. A researcher notes: "Patients' hypnotic recall of painful pressure to the head during birth is often enough to eliminate symptoms of chronic headache, including migraine. Cheek's patients commonly relate their reported birth experiences to present moods and behavior patterns. Many patients with asthma and emphysema were nearly suffocated during birth."[61] Understanding that *that was then, this is now,* helps these people change seedthoughts that are causing present-day distress.

Faith

Faith is accepting things unseen. It is believing without initial proof. Acting on a belief is evidence of faith! The proof or evidence people seek often comes after acts such as meditating, praying, chanting, visualizing or affirming. Anointing with oil, lighting a candle, and rain dancing are also actions people take to express their faith in something beyond themselves. They express one's faith in a higher power. Acting on faith may be the first prerequisite for healing yourself.

It's important to recognize that not everyone will heal themselves without medical intervention. Not everyone is meant to be released from illness in that way. Illness is a growth and learning process. Some are healed without drugs or surgery. For others, these medical interventions are an important part of the growth process. Roberta Tager observes, "Now we have medicine, surgery, assorted body therapies and love—perhaps the most important treatment there is. To quote my doctor husband, 'Spiritual healing can work hand in hand with medicine. It's another alternative.'"

A Zen monk once observed, "Healing begins in the mind." Faith in those words led my friend Martin to the attitude and behaviors that released him from cancer of the spinal cord. Even without the remission of cancer, he became a happier person.

Without some measure of faith most people wouldn't take the time to meditate, chant or do affirmations and visualizations. Faith plants life-affirming seedthoughts. If you are looking for ways to improve your life, *then you already have sufficient faith in a better future to do what it takes to create it.*

Self-Help Experience #37
Silent Sitting Meditation

Purpose: To improve your experience of meditation. Ananda Saha, a
Connecticut artist and meditation teacher, suggests the following guidelines for
sitting meditation:

1. It is important to take the commitment to meditate seriously. Regard the
   space you sit and practice in, as a sacred space.
2. Sitting practice is a time when you don't do anything else but try to apply
   clear comprehension. You simply sit, breathe and practice awareness with
   the goal of growing awareness.
3. Be aware that you are in a particular place: sitting, breathing, thinking and
   feeling. The more you learn to be aware of when you are drifting off or
   spacing out, the more you can apply clear comprehension, clear seeing of
   what simply is.
4. This awareness begins to expand into your post-meditation experience and
   even into times of crisis.

Self-Help Experience #38
Chanting

Purpose: Relaxation; quieting the mind; using sound creatively
Instructions
1. Have a reverent attitude before you begin to chant.
2. Some people sit cross-legged, others kneel, some sit in a chair and others
   choose to stand.
3. You can chant any of the mantras mentioned in this book, aloud or silently.
   Some teachers believe you must chant aloud, at least part of the time. The
   sound then vibrates and the vibration produces the result.

Following are three chants I've used successfully:

     Om Namah Shivaya

     Nam Myoho Renge Kyo

     Om Ta Ma Ra Om.

When you chant Ta, think red. When you chant Ma, think blue. When you chant
Ra, think yellow, and when you chant Om, think white.

Chanting Your Own Affirmation
Recently during an MRI test to make sure my brain tumor had not recurred, I
found the banging noise of the test made it difficult to chant, meditate or pray.
So, I used an affirmation in step with the noisy rhythmic beat of the test, to chant
inwardly. I repeated over and over, "Relaxed and happy from head to toe,"
saying one word for each beat. This allowed me to focus my mind and keep

calm, preventing me from thinking thoughts like, "I can't stand this," thoughts which were waiting to emerge. I felt great when the test was completed. The tumor is gone!

Self-Help Experience #39
Linda Zelizer's Guidelines
For Self-Hypnosis and Creating Affirmations

Purpose: General information to help you create effective affirmations. To create the conditions you want to appear in your life. This simple but powerful technique makes change easier, by tapping into both the intuitive and rational sides of your brain.

The subconscious mind can be a garden where you plant seeds, or a weed field left to chance. An affirmation is a powerful pesticide, eradicating a harmful seedthought while allowing a desirable thought to grow and multiply. Outer conditions in your life reflect your inner reality, so willfully changing your inner reality produces good results. Focus your thoughts on specific intentions as an effective personal, or even political, change agent. Affirmations use words to guide you creatively toward the experience of well-being.

Affirmations can be repeated aloud, thought silently or even written out daily to reinforce the chosen programming you are offering your mental computer. Affirmations used with imagery are most effective. Some people draw pictures related to the intended result. Affirmations are self-instructions. Repeat them many times daily for several weeks in order to produce your desired result. Just as a magnet attracts metal, the thoughts you dwell in become the reality of your life. Right words, thoughts and action are needed for healing. Make these a part of your Operating Manual.

Instructions

1. Define something about yourself that you want to change. Describe specific ways you would act when you reach your goal.

2. Relax your body and your mind using any of the relaxation techniques described in this book.

3. After you reach the relaxed state, use Visualization to imagine yourself reaching your goal. Mentally create that picture in great detail until you see or feel yourself feeling happy, having already made the change.

   For example:

   To lose weight, see yourself thin.

   To be able to speak comfortably in front of a group, imagine yourself speaking there.

   To eliminate a tumor from your body, first imagine it disappearing and then see your body without it.

To improve your general level of health, imagine your body functioning in perfect health and harmony.

4. Design an affirmation which recognizes you at your goal. Use the present tense. For example:

I feel healthy and alive.

I concentrate effectively.

My tennis game improves daily.

I am stronger and healthier and more balanced each day.

Don't use the future tense, because it creates an inner mind program which says that you are not ready now. The present tense, in contrast, affirms your readiness and willingness to reach your goal now. Keep the affirmation positive with the emphasis on you at your goal now.

One man read about hypnosis and began to affirm to himself, "I am *not* hungry." He actually gained weight. Each time he told himself "I am not hungry," he focused his attention inside to see if he was hungry. He thought about hunger so often that he put conscious energy into being hungry. He told me that he was more hungry when he used an affirmation denying hunger than when he didn't think about hunger.

Telling yourself not to do something, you focus attention on the very thing you are avoiding, making it harder to avoid—try not to think about a pink elephant as you read this. The mind and imagination must focus on the positive goal.

The wording you use is very important. You must use statements that your conscious mind can accept. For example, suppose you choose to work on your level of prosperity. To create wealth you decide to affirm, "I am a rich woman." This would be a wonderful affirmation IF your conscious mind would believe the statement. If you are thousands of dollars in debt but affirm "I am a rich woman," your conscious mind might be thinking, "Oh yeah, who says you're rich, you're broke!" That would reinforce the negative state—a lack of prosperity. In order for Affirmations to work they must be *reasonable, believable and acceptable to the conscious mind,* lest the mind dismiss the affirmation as mere wishful thinking. The mind must hear an affirmation and really believe it could be true or become true.

5. Stay with the Positive Image Visualization and Affirmation that you have created for several minutes. In this relaxed state, allow yourself to feel good and enjoy the scenario. If you do not feel good with what you are doing, change your imaging until you do feel good. Strong feelings help to reinforce your beliefs. Strong negative feelings may keep you repeating the same negative behavior. Strong positive feelings will reinforce the positive behavior.

6. To return to normal awareness, take a long deep breath and gently bring yourself back to consciousness of your present day environment. Return to awareness with the good feelings you have created during your Self-guided Visualization.

Self-Help Experience #40
Dr. Emmet Miller's Guidelines for Visualization

Purpose: To create positive expectations and/or experiences

Instructions

1. Find a safe, quiet place and allow yourself to get into a deeply relaxed state.
2. Visualize yourself, in great detail, behaving as you would like, stressing the benefits. Use all your senses in this imagining.
3. Search for any resistances to the change you would like to make. Be ready to modify your goal or move toward it slowly. Sometimes we aren't ready to give up unwanted behaviors because the behaviors get us something we want, or something our unconscious mind thinks we want.
4. Picture challenges to your newly chosen response pattern, and every day rehearse the new ways you plan to respond to each challenge.
5. Each evening, review all the challenges you experienced during the day. Celebrate your successful responses by positively acknowledging yourself. Rehearse any ways you would like to respond differently.

Self-Help Experience #41
Biblical Scriptures As Affirmations

Purpose: To provide a Judeo-Christian perspective for your affirmations

Some people are comforted reading the Bible—a dynamic self-help process. God's words are seedthoughts that grow into positive core beliefs when memorized and repeated regularly. Evangelist Kenneth Copeland says that we take charge of our lives by taking complete charge of our tongues. The following verses are prescriptions for living, or promises from God.

A soft answer turns away wrath, but harsh words cause quarrels. (Prov. 15:1)
Reckless words pierce like a sword: but the tongue of the wise brings healing. (Prov. 12:18)
A soothing tongue is a tree of life: but perverseness in it crushes the spirit. (Prov. 15:4)
A cheerful heart does good like medicine, but a broken spirit makes one sick. (Prov. 17:22)
God is our refuge and strength, a tested help in times of trouble. (Ps. 46:1)
A relaxed attitude lengthens a man's life; jealousy rots it away. (Prov. 14:30)
The wicked man's fears will all come true, and so will the good man's hopes. (Prov. 10:24)

In those days when you pray, I will listen. (Jer. 29:12)
I will give you back your health again and heal your wounds, saith the Lord. (Jer. 30:17)
No, I will not break my covenant; I will not take back one word of what I said. (Ps. 89:34)
These are the blessings that will come upon you:
    Blessings in the city, Blessings in the field;
    Many children, Ample crops, Large flocks and herds;
    Blessings of fruit and bread;
    Blessings when you come in, Blessings when you go out. (Deut. 28:2-6)
I have said I would do it and I will. (Is. 46:11)

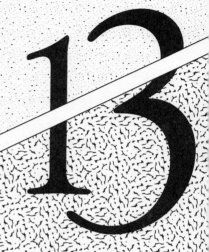

Dreamwork & Artwork

The Work of Bernie Siegel, M.D.

Through dreams you can communicate between your conscious and unconscious mind. This language connection uses symbols to take you to a space beyond your limited daytime awareness. The symbolism of the dream may initially escape your daytime mind's search for the meaning of your nighttime experience. Still, dreams are especially valuable because during sleep your conscious mind is turned down and its everyday judgments do not interfere. Then the dream can communicate what you need to know. You might get sick in an unconscious attempt to express your buried emotions. But through a dream you can rediscover and release stored emotional experiences in a helpful, healthful, benign fashion, making body illness unnecessary as a way of expressing emotions.

You can use sleep to heal yourself physically, emotionally, and spiritually. While dreaming you can work out fears, problems, negative emotions, and stressful relationships. These positive effects of sleep occur whether or not you remember dreaming.

Dreams provide you with an altered experience of reality, a different time and space reference. Scientific understanding of dream mechanisms is still in its infancy, though people have been turning to dreams for knowledge for centuries. Even the Bible speaks of prophecy divined through dreams.

The Metaphorical Language of Sleep

Here is an example of how I use my dreams. My "drilling dream" was short but very meaningful, and occurred on December 3, 1982.

"I dreamed Dr. Bernie Siegel was a dentist working on me. Drilling in my mouth, he works from left to right. I don't remember the work on the left, but he drilled a lot on my right. He had me open my mouth wide."

I wrote the following interpretation of the dream in my journal:

"I thought a lot about this dream, wondering about the meaning. Is this a message about health, or death? Dr. Siegel deals with cancer and death. I've listened to his taped lectures and read his written material. Though I've never really worried about cancer, I do fear illness and think about dying. The *right* side of my mouth is a dream symbol for my unconscious emotions just as the right brain represents the intuitive and unconscious. Dr. Siegel symbolically digs out my emotions, digging them out of solid rock (the tooth). Am I resisting the idea of death? Right now I believe drilling (to get at my cavities) is a symbol of the effort I must expend to make permanent changes in my attitudes and emotions. I also realize that I am indeed making those changes—one step at a time—and have been for years. The process will accelerate because now I have a *drill* to follow and excellent helpers to practice with."

After making my initial notes, I continued to try to understand this dream, which touched me deeply. Later I added the following: "Since the right side represents the unconscious, a dentist drilling there could be drilling into my subconscious to retrieve the knowledge that is stored there (drilling to remove). Or the idea behind the symbol of a dentist drilling could be a metaphor related to practicing a drill, of me drilling till I am master of the material and have learned my lessons. The dream metaphor thus relates to education in the original Latin sense of 'drawing out,' and education in the modern sense of cramming in. Drilling is a word with two meanings in this context. On the one hand, Dr. Siegel was my teacher, drilling information into me. On the other hand, he was drilling to retrieve information—my healing knowledge and experiences that I want to share in my book."

This drilling dream was significant and I immediately knew it. The dream gave me direction (leave what's left and go right/write). I had the dream six months before I began the first draft of this book. It confirmed what I would write (drill/retrieve/right) about. It also gave me the idea to ask Dr. Siegel and other professionals for help. Busy though he was, he gave me information, support, and encouragement.

Dreams can be prophetic. Two months after the drilling dream, I had dental work to remove an abscess on the root of a tooth on the *right* side of my mouth. This was the same spot where Dr. Siegel, as the dentist in my dream, was drilling. My bodymind, through the dream, prepared me for physical work I needed to help my body and save the tooth above the abscess.

Dreams Reveal, Not Conceal

During a workshop, Dr. Montague Ullman, psychiatrist, coauthor of *Working With Dreams* and founder of the Maimonides Hospital Dream Lab, provided some scientific background for my experience of dreams. He said:

> Dreaming is an activity we engage in regularly, during a profoundly altered state of being (as a natural part of the sleep cycle). The dream is a function of the waking state. When we waken we pull back part of the experience of dreaming. Pulling back and remembering the dream is an attempt to communicate, through language, an experience which has occurred in a different mode, a pictorial mode. The initial dreaming experience undergoes a transformation. During the process some information is lost.

> During dreaming we produce lots of imagery. The brain is programmed to generate images every 90 minutes. That is, we begin to dream whether we remember the dream or not. This has been determined by years of laboratory research with many different subjects. Dreaming is a universal phenomenon which should and could be accessible to all. Dreams are important communications we aren't paying enough attention to.

> *The purpose of the dream is to reveal, not conceal.* We rearrange visual images to express feelings we are experiencing at the time.

> Expressed in this manner they have an emotional impact. Metaphors are comparisons between two different things that reveal an underlying identity more powerfully than through the ordinary use of language. Dreams are visual metaphors and sometimes metaphors are difficult to understand. Sometimes ideas about the meaning of a dream come after the lapse of some time. In many instances, on awakening our dreams at first seem rather puzzling. Yet dreams shed light on our current life situation by helping us view the present from the perspective of the past. From that perspective, we may anticipate some things about the future, but we can't know the future. Dream work is healing in the sense of making us feel more whole.

Dr. Ullman recommends working on dreams with another person or group of people. I have sometimes found this helpful. The questions others ask on hearing about a dream, and the feedback the sharing generates, have been invaluable in my quest to know myself. The dream often re-arranges content from your current life within a new context. The altered perspective helps you view the present creatively. Don't talk about all your dreams, only those with such powerful imagery that they affect you emotionally. You will know the dreams whose meaning and metaphors need to be explored. Trust your intuition to lead you. Important dream messages will be repeated in different ways, until you get the message.

Interpret Dreams with Caution

Sometimes dreams foretell serious illness, or even death, for yourself or another. Dreams are then a helpful warning system. But because the dream is couched in symbolism and metaphor, the meaning can be unclear. Death dreams—subject to misinterpretation which increases fear—often don't relate to death at all. Sometimes dreams of illness or even death symbolize emotional processes that need exploration and healing. Don't take each scary dream literally. Dreams must be viewed in the context of a total life situation for a clear meaning to emerge.

Often death dreams have spiritual or emotional significance and indicate a change in the way the dreamer relates to the one who supposedly died. A teenager about to leave home or a woman wanting more independence from her husband might dream of a death in the family. Prior to leaving for college, my daughter Jennifer dreamed of my death on two occasions, which was at first frightening to me. But the date she gave came and went quite a while ago, and I am still here. From a metaphysical point of view, dreaming of a parent's death is a way for adolescents to deal with the process of growing up and detaching from the parent. Dreams of your own death can signify rebirth into a new way of being. Perhaps a new, more appropriate behavior is about to be established with death to the old behaviors.

The beauty and difficulty of dreamwork is that messages come in symbolic form. If you think your dream means some trouble is brewing in your life, take heed. Perhaps the dream was meant to alert you to a problem which can be avoided by appropriate action, like the action Pharoah took in the Biblical story of Joseph, when he stored grain in anticipation of famine.

J. Allan Hobson, a Harvard Medical School professor, is using student's dreams to acquaint them with the nature of another altered state—the psychotic experience. He said, "You can't hear it through a stethoscope and you can't see it on an X ray. Furthermore, patients are reluctant even to give you a description of it. But we regularly experience in our dreams, mental states more similar to psychosis than anything a patient, or I could describe in words." Hobson said that "every symptom of major mental illness is experienced in students' own dreams—disorientation, memory loss, bizarre thoughts, hallucinations, grandiosity, delusions and intense fear, rage and euphoria."[62]

There is some evidence for a new kind of dream called a "breakthrough dream." According to psychologist Joseph Hart, clinical director at the Center Foundation in Los Angeles, "It's a lucid, powerful dream. The dreamer has full feeling and expression. There's vivid, total recall of the dream, and it invariably has a strong therapeutic impact on the dreamer. Lee Woldenberg, the center's medical director, described the dream as a bridge between the power, feeling, and creativity of the unconscious mind and the clarity and cognitive abilities of the conscious mind. We're impressed with the psychotherapeutic potential of this kind of dreaming and are developing ways to teach people to dream this way." Besides help in healing oneself, dreams are reputed to have been involved in "breakthrough discoveries" in diverse fields of human endeavor, from scientific discoveries to ways of implementing new knowledge for the good of mankind.[63]

Above all, relax. Enjoy your dreams. Often, they are as interesting as a good movie. Psychotherapist Dr. Stephen Aizenstat is an authority on dreamwork. He says, "Feces are one of the most engaging images. Feces are manure, manure means seeds, seeds mean growth. When feces appear in dreams. I get hopeful. Right around the corner there's fertile ground for growth, new possibilities."[64] Dreams help shape reality.

Dr. Bernie Siegel, author and surgeon, is a former assistant clinical professor at Yale Medical School. Dr. Siegel has helped innumerable people with potentially fatal illnesses learn to live better and longer. These people, with cancer and other life-threatening illnesses, participate in Exceptional Cancer Patient (ECAP) groups with other exceptional patients. Each one is willing to take an active part in, and responsibility for, his or her own healing. The writings describe a remarkable force: the healing power of Love.

This smiling man, with the clean-shaven head, makes use of the dreams and drawings of his patients in the diagnosis and treatment of illness. His thesis is that spontaneous drawings, at critical moments in a person's life, are quite meaningful. As a surgeon, he can verify the diagnosis made on the basis of a patient's drawings. There appears to be a remarkable correlation between the intuitive diagnosis and the actual diagnosis, verified through medical/surgical techniques. It seems that the patient always knows, at some level of consciousness, what is going on in his body. The drawings are a way of moving past the conscious mind (which doesn't know), to the subconscious (which reflects its knowing in the drawings). Dreams serve the same function.

Dr. Siegel contends that patients, especially those with catastrophic illnesses, know the cause and course of their illness, at a deep unconscious level. They can retrieve this information through their dreams and drawings. If they are to alter the course favorably, change must occur at this level. Dr. Siegel recounts the following fascinating experiences with dreams:[65]

Dreams and Spontaneous Drawings

By Bernard S. Siegel, M.D. and Barbara H. Siegel, B.S.

Physicians are generally trained as mechanics, with very little attention paid to the relationship between psyche and soma. Due to a personal search and growth process, as well as a congenial relationship with Elisabeth Kübler-Ross, I was exposed to the work of Susan Bach, an English psychotherapist and student of Carl Jung. Susan's work with spontaneous drawings led to my own.

As a practicing surgeon, I explored the active role of the mind in illness and was astonished at the information available via dreams and drawings. I became aware that patients knew their diagnoses. The mind literally knew what was going on in the body. When I shared my beliefs and was open, the patients began to share with me their knowledge of the future events and the outcome of their diseases and treatments. Now I routinely ask for dream material and for drawings as part of their care and as part of the diagnostic testing process.

Dreams

A patient with breast cancer reported a dream in which her head was shaved and the word "cancer" written on it. She awakened with the knowledge that she had brain metastases. No physical signs or symptoms appeared until three weeks had passed, when the dream diagnosis was confirmed.

Another patient had a dream in which a shellfish opened and a worm presented itself. An old woman points and says, "That's what's wrong with you." The patient, a nurse, sick with an undiagnosed illness, awakens with the knowledge that hepatitis is her diagnosis. Her physician confirmed the diagnosis.

I Turn to Drawings

In view of my own limitations as a dream analyst, I have turned to drawings, which like the unconscious material in dreams, can be interpreted for diagnosis and appropriate therapy. Guidelines created by Susan Bach, assist in the drawing interpretation. Drawings have accurately predicted the time, and cause, of death.

Remember I am dealing with many severely, sometimes terminally, ill patients.

I ask patients to draw or symbolize themselves, their disease, their treatment, and their white blood cells. Then a new realm of information is presented to us. The dreams and drawings reveal the vital nature of our life processes. It is not only our emotions which come to the surface symbolically, but also our somatic and intuitive processes.

In drawing one's self, or using symbols of the self, such as birds, trees, or houses, we portray our unconscious knowledge of present and future. A quite sick four-year-old, draws a purple balloon floating up into the sky, with her name on it. There are multi-colored decorations around the balloon, plus a shape which resembles a cake. This child died on her mother's birthday.

A young man with a brain tumor (whose recent tests were all negative) drew a tree that looked exactly like the profile of a brain. The tree showed black throughout, suggesting to me recurrent cancer, which was subsequently detected by CAT scan.

Predicting the Results of Treatment

The future results of chemotherapy and surgery can also be revealed in drawings. If patients see their treatment as an insult, assault, or poison, they react accordingly, often suffering side effects. On the other hand, the unconscious mind which believes in and accepts the therapy, alters the side effects and produces a better therapeutic result. This information is important so that we may alter any negative beliefs before treatment.

One patient drew X ray therapy as black and red arrows spraying his body. He had a terrible reaction to the therapy. The drawing represented a negative expectation and the patient's belief was fulfilled.

Another patient drew X ray therapy as a golden beam of energy. This patient had an excellent result with no side effects. The drawing represented a positive self-fulfilling prophecy. This patient had peace of mind which presaged healing. 'Scientific' changes occur in the body when we have peace of mind.

Improving the Effects of Treatment

One of the most significant examples was a man who left his doctor's office when he was told the treatment would kill his cancer. He was a Quaker, a conscientious objector, and never killed anything. His drawing had been of little men carrying away his cancer cells. He is alive several years later, using his mind and vitamin C as healing agents.

An important point to be aware of is the difficulty our mind/body encounters as medicine wages a war on disease. The language of treatment is often depressing to the patient. Our bodies are the battleground, and the fact is that only a small percentage of people (15–20%) are comfortable being aggressive (killing the disease). The others manifest unconscious rejection of the treatment because of its association with destruction and killing. Physicians need to present the treatment as an aid to the healing process rather than as death to cancer or a war on disease.

Elisabeth Kübler-Ross emphasized the importance to me of "Thou shalt not kill" as a commandment in our conscious and unconscious minds. I have received drawings from patients with the cancer saying, "Help!" On other drawings the white blood cells look like popcorn so that they won't hurt the disease. The mind is aware that the disease is US.

I learned that we need to love ourselves in order to heal. The love stimulates our immune system, and white blood cells, to work for us. The effects of love and despair have been verified in studies of immune responses to various stimuli. We must learn to consume the disease by using it as nourishment... ingesting the disease as our white blood cells do, using it as a source of psychological growth. We learn ways to improve ourselves and love fully from disease. Disease leads to correcting an imbalanced pattern in the system. For some, disease can be seen as a healing of the soul.

Medical mechanics do not often realize the importance of patients' belief systems in the outcome of therapy. If we are to achieve *exceptional* results we must start working to unite the team of mind, body, and spirit. The dream process and visualization help us do this.

Dreams Guide Treatment

A patient listening to his inner voice often receives instructions via dreams or during meditation. One man who recovered, was asked to take injections of vitamin C and to utilize computer images for positive subliminal stimulation. Exploration of these techniques has just begun by orthodox medicine. It seems the inner voice preceded the medical profession in exploring the path to self-healing, or participation with the physician.

A woman was in severe pain and was told by a voice (she called it the Holy Spirit) that she had appendicitis and had better go to the Emergency Room. She said that she wanted to wait, but the voice insisted she go. My diagnosis simply confirmed her pre-existing knowledge.

As I have explored the nature of healing and have moved further from the mechanistic medical model, principles have arisen tying together many so-called mystical events. The body is not a machine but is a vibrant system of physical and electrical energy whose tissues and organs have their own frequencies and cycles, their own rhythms. The nervous system becomes the transmitter of this information to the conscious mind.

When a salamander loses a limb or a tail it is aware of the loss and it communicates with the injured part. It "listens" to the nerves in that area and answers by initiating regeneration.

Disease states represent an alteration in the pattern within the human energy system. If one "listens," the symptoms present themselves. For some, these symptoms, or this awareness, is through physical signs. But for many, the message comes via dreams, intuition, and the unconscious or spontaneous drawings which can be interpreted.

When I began to utilize the picture drawing technique in my surgical practice, I was able to see within the drawings the intimate relationship between psyche and soma. Also revealed to me was invaluable information stemming from the unconscious and from the individual's intuitive awareness.

In summary, may I say, that this exposure has led me to believe that the psyche and soma are communicating and that somatic problems can be brought to consciousness via symbols. Also, I believe as Carl Jung did, that "the future is unconsciously prepared long in advance and therefore can be guessed by clairvoyants."

These experiences have shown me a new path as a healer, teacher, care giver, and have reinforced my beliefs. My patients now feel free to share experiences they would never share with a mechanistic M.D.—one who sees only the mechanical process of disease in the body, without recognizing the totally integrated role of the mind and emotions.

Self-Help Experience #42
To Sleep, To Dream, To Remember

Purpose: To help in remembering your dreams

Instructions

1. You can improve your ability to remember dreams. Suggest to yourself at bedtime that you will recall a dream upon arising. "I intend to remember a dream." Remembering is a choice you make. Forgetting is also a choice, a choice that perhaps you have forgotten you made.

2. If you have a specific situation you are working on, before going to sleep *ask for guidance* related to that problem.

3. Keep a pencil and paper by your bedside to make note of any thoughts or images upon awakening. Allow time to wake slowly in the morning. If you recall a dream, tell yourself about it, to anchor it in your memory. Then write it down.

4. If no dream images or memories arise, notice what you are thinking about. Write down your thoughts. They might not be of a dream, but your night-time experiences will have led to your awakening thoughts which may or may not be useful to you. Take your dream journal with you if you leave home in the morning. Sometimes a dream is remembered later on.

5. If you still have trouble remembering a dream, think back to the last dream you remember having and try to analyze that. Often discovering an old dream's hidden meaning will enable you to move on to a new area in your life, with a new sequence of dreams.

6. Remember, you are the maker of the meaning in your life. A dream symbol may be meaningful to you alone. It's up to you to find any significant connections between your thoughts, your dreams, and your daily life. Not all dreams have significant meaning.

Self-Help Experience #43
How to Work with Dreams

Purpose: To improve the benefits you receive from your dreams, explore the meaning of a dream through questions you ask yourself. Questions help you to discover what present life context shaped the dream. If you know how the dream relates to your present life you may learn about changes in your life that are necessary. The relationship of a dream to your present life isn't always easily accessible. But those vivid dreams that are filled with shocking or stimulating imagery, generally have meaning that you can discover and use.

Sometimes it's helpful to share the dream with another person to get another impression. Often the reactions of the listener shed light on the meaning of a dream. At times, I've found my dream means more to my listener than to me. Once I dreamed of bodies piled on railroad cars. The reaction of the therapist I shared it with was much stronger than my own. Another time I dreamed about a man I'd worked with having his legs blown off during the war. That message, meant for both of us, was: "Being forced to your knees is a symbol of humility." Sometimes we might actually be dreaming for other people's benefit.

There are books written about the universal meaning of various symbols. Trust your intuitive voice to tell you what your symbol means to you. You'll know when you've made the right interpretation by the reaction of your body. Perhaps you'll get a tingle or some other felt-sense announcing a perfect fit. For in-depth work, join a dreamwork group.

Instructions

1. Trust yourself! Make a commitment to work with your dreams, and your internal wisdom will guide you into understanding the message.

2. Write down your dream and give it a title.

3. Notice any striking images and ask what they might mean. Pay special attention to recurring images, be they people, animals, places, or things.

4. Ask yourself, "What current event in my life is connected to this dream?"

5. Ask yourself, "What is this dream trying to tell me?"

6. Wait several hours or even a few days and then re-read what you wrote. Sometimes you will have forgotten the original dream. Then your written words are often more meaningful. Sometimes, my dream means nothing to me until I read what I wrote and then it almost seems like a direct message for me to do something. For example, I might write down, "I was traveling on the right road." Those kinds of notes confirm what I am doing in life.

7. As you re-read your dream notes, pay attention to any thoughts you are having. Inspirational messages often come while re-reading dream notes.

Go the distance
Honesty is the best policy
Think for yourself

Creating a New Context:
Healing From Within

14

In chronic or recurrent acute illnesses your lifestyle is often key to your state of health. Lifestyle includes how you language your life: your attitude, thoughts, emotions, and style of thinking. You can create conditions more favorable to health by removing unhealthy negative belief systems. To be permanently effective, healing must occur in the mind.

The body acts out thoughts and images. Usually you aren't aware of this process in much the same way that you aren't usually conscious of breathing and other automatic body functions. But just as you can bring consciousness to bear on the process of breathing (choosing to breathe deeply, for example), you can positively influence many aspects of your body when you choose to pay attention.

Why Am I Sick? Because...

When thoughts and images are consciously chosen, the mind can create a context for health. A context is a frame of reference, a milieu, or an environment within which you operate. To recognize your present context, pay attention to those "why" questions you ask yourself, and listen to the different

169

"becauses" you answer. Notice too your "why nots," "buts," and "if onlys." These connect to beliefs about the way things *should be* for us to be happy. The "becauses" are beliefs about what makes people sick. These beliefs can be harmful. Your health context contains all the beliefs that keep those "becauses" in place. Many of the contextual beliefs that can harm you are buried in your unconscious. Asking "why" can bring them out and lead to more aware behavior.

Do you believe something will happen to you if you sleep less than eight hours, if you don't use rain gear, if you eat so-called junk food? Then perhaps you do need to get enough sleep, wear a raincoat and boots and eat better. Does the missed sleep or the lack of raingear or the junk food make you sick or do your beliefs about them cause you to be sick? Not everyone gets sick when they don't get enough sleep or when they get their feet wet or when they eat so-called unhealthy foods. Most people believe what they see. But, you will often see it because you already believe it. Healing from within requires you to discover what you already believe and how those beliefs affect you.

You can reduce the power of harmful beliefs and create a more favorable health context by using affirmations. For example, "I am generating health because I say so" puts healing forces in motion. I created a favorable context for my own healing by continually affirming, "I am grateful to my pure and perfect body for all it teaches me."

Shelly Bruce, one of the stars of the musical *Annie,* was happy and successful. Then, suddenly she was diagnosed as having leukemia. In her book, *Tomorrow Is Today,* she describes her illness and provides an example of altering context. During her difficult hospitalization she was playing the part of victim to the hilt, while slowly being destroyed by forces she felt were beyond her control. Eventually, she realized that as a performer there was another way to play her life/role. She could play it like Annie, be master of her fate, and emerge triumphant.

Shelly created a new context when she said she was no longer a victim and chose to be an optimist. She rejected her fear and embraced a more positive future, one filled with hope. Her faith was quickly rewarded when she received her first visible sign of improvement—no leukemia cells after her next bone marrow test.

She created a more positive *context* in which to hold the *content* of her life, which was her case of leukemia. As I write this, Shelly Bruce is free of leukemia and again performing. A miraculous beneficial side effect of her transforming self-improvement work was improvement in her singing voice. The transformation she experienced is available to you. "Miracles" are natural occurrences to those with faith and health-producing belief systems.

Since we do learn from adversity, that which seems to block us from our fervent desires may actually be there for our highest good. Sometimes we have lessons to be learned and knowledge of the self to gain before we can be healed. I now see benefits in my own prolonged healing before and after brain surgery. Learning patience and faith was a blessing. Learning to release envy and self-pity were gifts to myself—all growth resulting from my tumor.

After I was released from the hospital, while still unable to drive, I saw my friend Pat. She had had a mastectomy several weeks earlier and had to be concerned about the cancer recurring. But she was up and around and really seemed fine, while I was still struggling, walking with a cane, barely able to focus my eyes, unable to talk above a whisper. I envied Pat and felt very sorry for myself.

Several months later Pat's cancer recurred. She developed brain cancer and suffered many of the symptoms I had. I quickly realized the futility of envy. Pat died a difficult death from cancer a year after that "pity party" I held for myself. And years later, I am still alive and doing well. Pat taught me a profound truth: Don't envy anyone. You never know what they will have to bear. Just be grateful for what you have.

Tumors

Dorothy Thau is a holistic health counselor who supports her patients in healing from within, teaching them to alter unhealthy contexts by recognizing and changing seedthoughts and core beliefs. She recounts this story:

I had a 42-year-old patient with non-malignant intrauterine tumors. After fourteen months they were the size of a four-month pregnancy. This patient wanted to know why she had the tumors.

In the first session I taught her visualization using guided imagery. During the session she was surprised to see the growths not as tumors but as an embryo, as if she was creating another child. She realized that subconsciously she felt that she had never completed her duty as a female. She would have liked to have had more children. The connection between her desire and the uterine problem surprised her. At last she understood her emotional connection to the tumors. She needed to forgive herself and release her guilt feelings related to 'no more children.'

During her second session, I gave her these affirmations to use during her daily visualizations: 'My love and commitment to children can be fulfilled through my teaching career, as well as through my own two children. The job of my uterus is complete and it can relax and stop trying to create anything new.' She left with tools to alter her negative beliefs, feeling relieved and more relaxed."

Another of Dorothy Thau's patients, a 56-year-old woman with diabetes used insulin daily.

Her goal was to halt the progression of her illness. During our work her circulation and eyesight improved and her use of insulin was drastically reduced.

A breakthrough occurred after a treatment session where we used Age Regression Therapy. I regressed her eleven years to the onset of her disease, coinciding with her divorce from her husband. She recalled, 'I felt the *sweetness* had gone out of my life.' She then saw the connection between her illness, diabetes, and her emotions surrounding the divorce.

She made rapid progress as she worked at letting go of any negative feelings about her ex-husband and the divorce. She affirmed, 'I feel positive about myself and my talents. I can live a sweet and fruitful life, in perfect health.'

After completing the treatment, her personality changed. She is now in terrific shape. A prolific artist and art teacher, she puts in long hours and smiles continually. The sweetness has returned to her life! Previously, she had thought of herself as a 'diabetic,' living with that label, seeing herself as diseased and disabled. She no longer considers herself limited or diseased, certainly a dramatic *reversal of the context* in which she previously saw herself.

According to Bridgeport endocrinologist Dr. Bob Lang, "People with diabetes often express the perception that 'there is no sweetness in life.' That thought is often stress-inducing. Recurrent negative thoughts may be responsible for triggering illness or worsening an existing disease condition."

Researchers at the University of Pittsburgh are studying the effects of shocks on the immune system. They report that there is often an association between the onset of diabetes (the content) and a separation, divorce, or the death of a parent (the context).[66]

Backbone

Linda Zelizer treated a woman with severe back problems who chose to explore the related emotional components. She remembered the words her mother used frequently before her death. "When I die, I want you to be the backbone of this family." She was already feeling pressured in her life. She did not want to be "the backbone" of her family. She realized that while she had always had some back problems, their severity increased dramatically when her mother died.

She found it easier to use her physical problems to avoid unwanted tasks than to say "No" and deal with the consequences. The payoff for her ill-health was avoidance of responsibilities. Understanding the relationship of her physical distress to the seedthought "be the backbone of the family" led her to change her behavior, thus easing her backache problems.

But Zelizer says, "I've seen many cases where a payoff or secondary gain is an obstacle to the patient's getting well, and might be the reason for the unwanted behavior in the first place. Patients usually aren't aware of this payoff. Sometimes people come for hypnosis to change a specific habit and a deeper, underlying issue surfaces. Although they want to change the habit at one level, they are not always willing to deal with the deeper level. Sometimes they have some emotional investment in not solving the problem. Hypnosis is a wonderful tool but it is not magic."

Another Zelizer patient was a young boy with recurrent ear infections and difficulty in hearing. He told Zelizer that he often said to himself, "I don't want to listen to you" when thinking about his verbally abusive father. They explored ways he could handle his father's put-downs. The boy learned to assert himself by telling his father "I don't like what you say." He used his imagination to create his relationship with his father getting better. He realized that his father's treatment of him related to the father's own bad feelings about himself. The new payoff was far fewer ear infections and improved hearing.

The Authentic You

Dr. Bernie Siegel's approach to healing is partly based on the concept that people's illnesses result from living lives that are not in accord with their authentic selves. Then conflict, stress, and negative emotions that disrupt the body's ability to control disease are generated. Fortunately, when people begin to act authentically, they can often reverse the process. Dr. Siegel helps people—with so-called fatal illnesses as well as "serious/chronic" ones—learn to live better and longer. Life-threatening becomes life-enhancing as he teaches patients how to achieve peace of mind and better health by understanding and loving themselves. Dr. Siegel uses the orthodox medical tools, from surgery to chemotherapy, to remove cancer. But he knows that a dose of loving attention, from oneself and others, is a powerful healing force.

To create a health-ful context and effect inner healing, it is helpful to know what the patient unconsciously believes about his illness and its recommended treatment. Bernie's patients' drawings are a vital element in the healing process. Often the material gleaned from drawings leads to an alteration of the dis-ease context. If the drawings reveal their perception of the treatment to be an attack, they often suffer side effects. So he first works with them on reversing negative information stored in the unconscious.

This change of context, from focusing on the outer manifestations of disease to looking at the inner perceptions, has totally changed Siegel's life. It has given him a renewed sense of fulfillment in his profession, as well as vastly increasing his impact on his patients, and his influence on the general public through his best-selling books. By discovering his own authentic self, he has pointed thousands of others towards discovering the authenticity of themselves.

Creating a Health-Full Context

Many years ago, President John F. Kennedy created a context for the success of the United States space program by *saying* that the U.S. was committed to a man walking on the moon in ten years. Kennedy gave his word when he created that commitment for all of us—to put a man on the moon. To regain and maintain good health requires commitment too. Take a stand! Give your word! Promise to work towards good health! Giving your word is evidence of your commitment to your goal, a big part of the language connection. *You* make the agreement, a promise to fulfill, a resolution you will keep. Love and accept yourself. Be alert to the process without attachment to the end result. If you learn from your experience, you are always a success, never a failure.

I have a context for my life that is large enough to include many aspects—self-confidence, worry, negativity, a positive outlook, joy, sorrow, pain, limitations, illness, and health. I attempt to make the most of each day. Sometimes I worry about various bodily sensations, but I always believe that essentially I am okay. Helpful images are those that represent life the way we want it to be. Images of suffering may be useful warnings, but aren't valuable as places to dwell. Since we attract to us that which we dwell on, I pay attention to warnings of doom, but dwell on positive, uplifting, health-producing images. When I relax and stop worrying about my bodily sensations, I feel and see myself healthier, and often become my good health.

Roberta Tager sums up what I believe inner healing is all about. She says, "I believe that the sole reason for bodily discomfort is so that our soul may learn. My body is the vehicle for my soul. Learning can take place at a very rapid rate. When one walks through life with an eye for the whole, one can step gently and correct each wrong step quickly. We each have chosen our lessons, only we have forgotten that we chose them.

"The enslavement of my soul has ended, and the learning and growth I chose is now available to me. Understanding attitudinal lessons is my way to release illness. The answer always lies within easy reach through meditation. Wellness is the natural state of the body. Releasing faulty thoughts allows wellness to return. This in no way negates the helpfulness of medical, surgical, or nutritional assistance."

True healing means knowing that ultimately we all die, and that during our life we will each face trials and tribulations. True healing is living within your circumstances and learning every step of the way. True healing is going through the process awake, aware, alert, with acceptance, love, and joy. True healing means living your life as both actor and audience: the performer and the objective observer each can enjoy the show. True healing is concerned with the *experience,* not attached to the *end result.* If it works and an illness is reversed or a life saved, great! If not, at least you know you "made the most of it."

Self-Help Experience #44
Writing Yourself to Wholeness

Purpose: To keep track of experiences, uncover emotions, materialize what you want, and avoid what you don't want

Instructions

1. Write your feelings in your journal. Notice what makes you happy and what makes you feel upset. Write down any discoveries you make about yourself, i.e., I found out I feel happier all day if I get up early and start working, even though I prefer to sleep late in the morning.

2. Awfulize and catastrophize any problem by imagining and writing down the worst that can happen. See how absurd the worst case is. Cross it out. Laugh it away.

3. Record your dreams.

4. List goals for a week, a month, three months, one year, five years, and ten years. Goals can be specific to fitness and health. For example:

    I will lose 25 pounds this year.

    I will improve my cardiovascular system by decreasing my resting pulse 10 beats.

    Include goals that support your psychological health as well. These could relate to work, relationships, and money, among others.

5. Choose a specific health-related area to work on. Write an affirmation regarding that area.

Self-Help Experience #45
Visualization for Strengthening the Immune System

Purpose: To rid your body of unwanted organisms

The immune system contains white blood cells patrolling the body through the blood and lymphatic systems. There are two main types: T cells, produced in the thymus gland, are killer cells which destroy invading bacteria and viruses; B cells, produced in the bone marrow, neutralize poisons made by disease organisms while helping the body mobilize its own defenses. The immune system is controlled by the brain, either directly through the nerves and neurochemicals or indirectly through hormones in the bloodstream. Immunological changes can take days or weeks, unlike many other autonomic or hormonal changes that can take seconds or minutes.

According to one theory, cancer cells often appear in the body and are destroyed by white blood cells before they grow into dangerous tumors. When the immune system becomes suppressed and can no longer deal with this routine threat, cancer or some other disease might develop. So too, if the brain's control of the immune system is compromised, ill health might follow. Conversely, whatever strengthens your brain's control of your immune system will probably improve your health.

In this exercise, you send a symbolic warrior to stimulate your immune system and aid your white blood cells in ridding your body of any intruding organisms. Use this for any infection, allergy, growth, or tumor. Some immune-enhancing agents might be white knights, doctors in white coats, Pacmen, polar bears, warfare weapons, vehicles like tanks or garbage trucks, squirt guns, and the letters T and B. You might like to use weapons of love, like valentines, or a laser beam of golden light.

Instructions

1. Relax into the helpful alpha state.

2. Choose your helper symbol and imagine it traveling throughout your entire body. Imagine it removing any unwanted organism.

3. When you are finished, thank your helper for the work it did. Tell yourself, "This process strengthened my immune system."

4. Practice this with eyes closed, seated or lying down. When you get good at this you can do it with your eyes open.

Self-Help Experience #46
Changing Attitudes

Purpose: To leave an unwanted situation without self-righteousness; to uncover your beliefs and change your attitude

Instructions

1. People often make another person or thing wrong, in order to justify their current point of view. This self-righteous thinking often leads to hostile words and harmful behavior.

   For example, people often bad-mouth a relationship that they want to leave. They attack the other person in their thoughts and words. This leads to continuing hostility and angry feelings.

   There is no need for you to attack that which isn't right for you in order to leave. You don't have to justify what you do by harming someone else. There may be some situations where it is necessary to present your point of view about another, but in general this isn't necessary. More helpful languaging is to think and/or say, "This situation/relationship is not appropriate for me right now. I choose not to be here."

2. Pay attention to the reasons you give yourself for doing what you do. Evaluate the usefulness of thinking that way. Notice how your thoughts lead to your current attitudes. If you want to change your attitude, choose more appropriate thoughts.

Self-Help Experience #47
The Daydreaming Exercise: Imaging to Help the Planet

Purpose: To change your thinking and change your world

We affect our health, as individuals, through the metaphors and beliefs evident in the stories that we tell ourselves. We can imagine sickness or we can imagine health.

In the same way, images and metaphors shared by members of a group, an organization, or a culture have a profound effect upon the group as a whole, as well as individuals within the group. We can imagine war, or we can imagine peace. You can imagine a worst case or a best case scenario. It's your choice.

Spend time imagining the whole world being the way you want it to be.

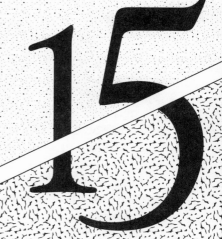

Make the best of it
Practice what you preach
Healer, heal thyself
Keep on keeping on

Keys to My Survival

"**W**hat did you do to survive your brain surgery? What did you think, feel, and believe that helped you? What gives you strength that might inspire me?" This chapter was written in response to a friend's questions in 1988, long after the original manuscript was first completed in 1984. Writing it has been hard, but nonetheless a real gift to myself, because I had to look deep within and codify my beliefs, learning a lot about myself during that difficult process.

I notice I'm more sure of myself and more clear about my opinions than ever before. I am clearer, too, about my language connections. Evidence continues to mount—from both my personal experience healing myself and my professional life researching and writing this book—for the existence of a mind/body link and the fact that language is a key connecting mechanism. When I am ill I look for connecting language and am often rewarded with my seedthought. The real inner me is more accessible now.

Healing Methods and Beliefs

My health continues to improve from the low level to

179

which it descended when I was thirty-two years old, fat, and lacking in energy. I have a brain scan each year to make sure the tumor hasn't recurred. (So far so good.) When I don't follow the rules I've learned for myself, mild illnesses often result. Perhaps my digestion acts up, or I'll have an occasional rash. Recently, I had a three-month episode of hypertension. When I am deeply concerned about something, my system responds with elevated pressure. But I've learned how to keep my blood pressure lower now. I live through each new experience, learn from it, and move on.

Writing this book was often more uncomfortable than I expected. When I had difficulty digesting or assimilating my experiences, I sometimes felt physically distressed. Then I used de-stressing techniques like meditation, affirmations, exercise, and massage. I also ate better. At times the only thing to do was to live through the discomfort, with as much non-judgmental awareness as I could muster. Often, the problem cleared up just by living through it and observing it with detachment.

My first chosen affirmation, repeated over and over again early on in my quest to help my physical body, was, "I give thanks for my pure, perfect, whole, and holy body." A massage therapist I used then also kept telling me how healthy I was.

At first I didn't believe it or her. My subconscious mind was invalidating the goal I was affirming by rebelling against the affirmation. I would say to myself, "What makes you think you are healthy?" But the therapist's positive belief about me and my practice affirmations worked well together. I soon realized that my body is a perfect vehicle for learning my life lessons, which made it easier to accept and give thanks for my perfect body. After a while I noticed how much better I was feeling. I found myself wholeheartedly affirming that I was indeed healthy and had a body that worked very well.

I reaffirmed my belief in *thinking for myself* and in self-induced healing. I began to understand what my *self* really is. My beliefs gave me the strength and will to survive the ordeal of brain surgery and the long recovery period.

Looking Ahead

I believe I am special and have a mission to accomplish. In 1985 I wrote a newsletter about my brain surgery. I shared it with hundreds of people. Sometimes I felt embarrassed when giving the letter to a stranger. But if I thought I should share it, I did. The response from many people was favorable. I think they were inspired by me, as I was inspired by them. The personal stories these people told me often helped me to feel better about myself and encouraged me to keep on keeping on.

I give meaning to the events in my life. I have a purpose. I chose to survive in order to complete my mission, part of which is to spread the information in this book.

I believe there is a Supreme Being, a God who guides and watches over me. I feel divinely protected. I have a personal relationship with that creative God force in the universe. That force is neither male nor female, but both. I say "Mother/Father/God" when I pray. I believe God created us all to receive His blessings. A belief in a Supreme Being is often rejected by people until they reach a crisis and discover the power of prayer and faith. Faith activates healing.

I expected people around me during my surgery and recovery period to get better as well. My attitude was, "If I have to suffer like this, then at least other people should benefit, making it more worthwhile for me." I was almost demanding that those around me improve themselves. Many did!

I believe I am responsible for myself and say this often. I have a team of doctors who advise and treat me. As the captain of my team I make the final decision based on expert advice. I trusted Dr. Dogali, my neurosurgeon, and during surgery he was in charge. I believed he could help me and had faith in his treatment. During my hospital stay, if I thought I needed something, I asked for it, sometimes quite forcefully. I fought for what I believed in. At least once, I was wrong. I admitted it.

During the early stages of my recovery I felt that I was proving myself and the message in this book. "Practice what you preach, Barbara, to learn what you teach." I believe each illness I have is part of my research. I take myself seriously. But, I also laugh at myself. I often told myself, "You are 'hot stuff' for having gone through brain surgery and survived to report on it." Perhaps the tumor and resultant surgery served to validate my whole existence at a subconscious level.

At times, I ask myself, "If you know so much how come you couldn't heal yourself without surgery? How come it's taking so long to fully heal? Why do you still have physical limitations? Why did you have to go through all this?" But the answer comes quickly, "Because going through all this taught you what you are sharing. Perhaps more importantly, your journey of tumor/growth/release allowed you the time and experiences you needed to change and improve yourself." The fact that things take time to resolve is truly the gift of time. When we see our tough experiences from the perspective of distance in time, we often perceive them as blessings in disguise.

I believe the main purpose of life is to learn. Life on Earth is like being in college. There are courses we take by attracting people and/or circumstances to learn from. We might not always like it. Perhaps we don't always choose the courses, but we do choose our receptivity to learning when the lesson appears. As part of the process, I use my body as a guide to uncover my emotions, thus learning from my body. Disease is a life-learning process, not necessarily a distinctive event.

I can sometimes choose what to experience and sometimes I must take what I get. Some things are unavoidable, predestined, written in stone. My tumor probably was. But we have some real choice. My growth from the tumor depended on choosing to learn from it.

I believe life has many goals. I choose my goals, which serve my life's lessons. I believed I would eventually reach my goal of better health and improved physical functioning, so long as I took each step necessary to complete the journey. I always keep my end goal in mind so the process is just what I have to do to get there.

A primary purpose of life is to have fun. A key to my survival is my keen interest in what happens, good or bad, and my belief that everything that happens to me is an adventure. While going through many of these adventures, I hate them or fear them and wish I could avoid them.

I believe we must play life like a game. I'm still learning to do this. As a game it is fun, but when I play it for real, I often suffer. It's funny, because I don't like the roller coaster, which many people ride for excitement. But, I guess one could say the roller coasters I get my kicks from are some of the problems I've had in life. Sometimes I even think the more the merrier. Cancel that thought!

I believe in the power of visualization, imagination, and prayer. I use these tools daily. I call a friend or a prayer line when I am really worried. I believe in the laws of agreement. An idea whose time has come depends on the agreement in principle of lots of people. Many people agreed with me and told me they believed I'd recover. That helped. Thoughts seem to get stronger the greater the number of people that believe in them.

Though I am Jewish, I believe in and often use the name of Jesus in my prayers. He was with me in the darkest times. Whenever I had a really tough experience to go through, I prayed, sometimes using the Lord's Prayer and sometimes the Twenty-Third Psalm, which I had memorized for just such tough times. At other times I inwardly chanted a mantra like "Om Namah Shivaya," or even made up an affirmation that was appropriate at the time. No matter what, I usually believed God was there with me, guiding my thoughts and actions.

I frequently "made believe" that I was better than I really was. I pretended to everyone, even myself. Pretending is the force that creates the new reality. Sometimes, I still pretend.

I believe in the probability of reincarnation. It makes sense to me that a loving God would allow us another chance to do it right, to make up for past mistakes. But I can't prove reincarnation. I don't believe that I am going to come back in this same body. But rather, the witness in me, the eye (I) watching me, experiencing my life and learning from it, will choose a new human form to return in, and learn some new lessons. Hopefully, it will be easier for me next time.

I believe the mind is like a tape recorder. We have memory tapes which often get stuck, so we replay them over and over. Yet we can erase the pattern of memories being replayed with the tools I've written about. The content of the unconscious part of your mind often affects you as much as the content of your conscious mind and maybe even more. So it's important to get to know the hidden you and work to change any harmful unconscious programming.

Sometimes I think I'd rather not be so aware. I don't want to know the future, but I'd still like to be prepared for diverse eventualities. Ignorance is not bliss, because at some point we will wake up to reality. I seem to believe in "Expect the best, prepare for the worst." I'm not yet sure whether that seedthought is good programming or not.

I have a purpose—to be a translator and transformer. Transformers wake people up, helping to activate love, faith, forgiveness and service to the highest self. Translators speak the language of and see the good in others, be they different religions, or groups like est that aren't religious, or even social movements like feminism. Different words often describe similar experiences and goals in different people. Translators help to synthesize divergent points of view by recognizing the common goals, purposes, and experiences of different people.

It may be easier to find fault rather than good in others, but it's not healing. There is power to heal ourselves and the planet in the concept of unity in diversity. That means we are one people, on planet Earth with many ways of expressing who we are and what and how we believe. But we are all connected and need one another to survive whether we are conscious of that fact or not.

I believe life is for-giving! I believe I awakened my inner strength when I committed myself, many years ago, to the idea of being of service in the world. At that time, I became President of the Connecticut chapter of the National Organization for Women and started teaching and lecturing about "thinking for yourself." I believe that what goes around comes around. Life can either be like a vicious circle or a golden ring. What you sow you reap. It's important for me to plant healthy seeds and to keep the soil of my life as free and clear and fertile as possible. It's important for me to give, and then I feel worthy to receive. Forgive and you shall be forgiven.

The past few years have been a period of intense questioning for me as I reflected on my fifteen-year quest to be free of the tumor. I explored the philosophies, the life and practices of different groups and religions, looking for healing alternatives. The tumor IS gone, but my search continues for ways to heal the damage to my nerves. I am still learning, growing, asking questions, testing beliefs, loving the process. I used to live by "making the best of it." Now I believe in "making the most of it." There is a difference.

One thing I strongly believe is that if we give people information and time, they will find the truth. As Phil Donohue often says, "Let's hear some wisdom from the audience." I believe each of you has the ability to think and discern what's right for your-self.

Illness or any crisis situation is a time of heightened potential. We may be more vulnerable, but then we have the chance to grow. As we say good-bye to the old ways, some part of us dies. You leave something you need to leave, in order to grow and move on. Perhaps a message of the great spiritual teachers from Buddha to Moses to Jesus is that there's no life without suffering and no joy without sorrow. What the Bible is telling us is that there is no promised land without an exodus, no resurrection without a crucifixion, no life without death; that is a part of human reality related to our spiritual journey.

Part of healing is learning to be comfortable with our emotions. The language of emotion is sparse, possibly a result of our difficulty handling emotions. Take the word "love." We have one word which we say to express the feeling of love for everything from food, to sex, to people. Surely we don't love each of these in the same way. We need new words to make distinctions between those different feelings of love. Learning to love and accept ourselves is basic to human education. So is learning to language emotion in a positive way. Ultimately when we learn to truly love and accept ourselves, we'll be able to live well and love each other and every thing we encounter.

I trust in serendipity, those accidental (?) happenings in life that might actually be God working for our highest good.

I think all healing ultimately stems from the mind. Sometimes we need to do something physical like take medicine or have surgery to support the mind's belief that healing will occur. We need external support because our minds aren't strong enough to believe the healing will occur without that physical crutch. The mind alone, a gift from God, could probably heal any condition but for our disbelief.

During the worst times, right after my brain surgery, when I was wheelchair-bound and unable to focus my eyes, I never lost hope. Deep inside, I always expected to get better. Prior to the surgery, I expected I'd be back to normal within a few months. I recently recognized a seedthought "I was ambushed." I was really surprised by how damaged I was. The degree of my difficulties caught me off guard, which could have easily led to despair. I had trouble even realizing what had happened to me. By the time it truly sank in how disabled I was, I had surrendered to the healing process. I'm changing the "ambush" programming.

I see now that my faith was very deep. Given my prior emotional track record and my typical pattern of worrying, I could have been in a panic. But in fact, I was too busy planning how to get well to spend time speculating that I might not recover. I used to think that I needed to worry in order to protect myself from some feared consequence or event. That belief is dissolving now.

Worry will not protect me from a disaster over which I have no control. If I feel a worry attack, where I am "awfulizing" by visualizing all kinds of unwanted occurrences, I turn to prayer to occupy my mind in a positive way. I use all the tools in this book and they help me. I believe in dwelling on best case scenarios, not worst case scenarios.

It is my dream that each reader of this book will continue the journey within, arriving at better health and a richer, more rewarding life. It is my hope that each of you will think for your self—that inner self—and recognize who and what that self really is. It is my hope that you will be committed to your path, a peace-path, not a war-path, and that you will have faith that your journey through life will bring you the rewards you each deserve.

Most of all, remember that you are not bad or wrong when you suffer pain or illness. You have illness to learn something. I believe that we attract the experiences we need in order to learn. But there is also a randomness to the events in the universe. We can be in the right place at the right time, or the wrong place at the wrong time. I believe we are not to blame. Responsibility means accepting what happens without self-reproach, guilt, self-hate, or negativity.

You don't have to be sick to get better! It takes courage to live life fully, exploring and experiencing all that is there for you. I applaud your persistence, even as I have applauded my own.

Test the principles in this book in your own life. Use the exercises in this book to help you become more aware—of how you think, what you feel, and what you say. Recognize the creative power of your words and thoughts and see how they contribute to your version of life. Accept only that information which you know is for your highest good. Ignore what doesn't help you.

Self-Help Experience #48
Starting a Support Group—The Bliss Group

Purpose: To start a group to support people who are okay and who love life

There are many groups that support people in times of trouble. Some are the anonymous groups like those serving alcoholics, drug addicts, child abuse victims, gamblers, etc. Other like ECAP (Exceptional Cancer Patients) serve those in a health crisis. Still other groups assist weight watchers or divorcees or widows. There seems to be a support group to help you through every kind of problem.

I believe everyone, in crisis or not, needs a loving support group. Social and religious organizations often provide this kind of support. I am a member of a very special group founded for the purpose of assisting each woman member in achieving a high-quality life and then spreading that good feeling to others. The key to the success of the participants in the Bliss Group is the affirmation each woman makes in order to join: "I am the Source of life showing up as Bliss. I am committed to the women's group for one year." Thus, each woman is the source of and responsible for her group's success.

My Bliss women's group meets once a month in a different member's home. The hostess sends a letter to each member sharing her vision for the evening and choosing a topic she would like each of us to address. We had 16 women in our group. But this idea is so powerful that three new groups formed from that original one. All together, there are about two hundred women committed to the Bliss group, a loosely structured network of women in New York and its suburbs who follow a monthly format similar to my group.

We have dinner, socialize, and usually speak on a specific topic chosen in advance by the hostess of the evening. There are two women who serve as resource for each group. My purpose as resource for my group is to assist the other members in whatever ways seem appropriate to me.

Sample Topics:

- How to achieve intimacy in relationships
- Loving ourselves and our bodies
- Managing money successfully
- Families: what are they, who are they?
- Friendships: meaning and purpose
- Integrity, trust, and authenticity

Sample Visions for the evening's outcome:

- Each woman will feel closer to other members of the group.
- We will each be more responsible for ourselves and take better care of our bodies.
- We will improve our ability to handle money.
- We will each be more aware of and accepting of our own feelings, rather than the beliefs and feelings we adopted from others.
- Our friendships will be deeper, richer, and more mutually supportive.
- We will experience our own integrity.

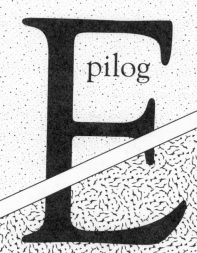

The tide has turned
Make light of it
Every dark cloud has a silver lining

Epilog

In the spring of 1988, I began re-editing this book under the guidance of my publisher, Dawson Church. Part of the process included updating the book to include a smattering of the latest research, especially in relation to the immune system. Since the events described in the Introduction to this book and the first draft of my manuscript, many books and articles have appeared supporting these ideas. Updating and revising is lots of work, and I'd never worked under such a limited deadline. Still, I joyfully welcomed the opportunity to complete my book's gestation and give birth to it.

I've been told that in writing a book and sharing one's own personal growth, a person often finds her difficult area in life "coming to a head." Problem areas can be faced, the experience digested, and the author is then released to grow into the next challenging space in her life. For example, when I finished the first draft, I found that I still had a tumor. I had surgery and was released from that rare growth. Still I was surprised by what happened as I finished the last draft. I had been feeling very strong and healthy. But I was "stewing" emotionally over difficulties involving a family-owned business run by my husband.

On May 3, 1989, (my daughter Jennifer's 19th birthday) I had a magnetic resonance imaging (MRI) exam of my skull. I thought it would be routine—if an MRI or CAT scan can ever be considered routine. It was an integral part of my yearly checkup to ensure that I remained tumor free.

On May 4, I was told that something unforeseen was discovered. I spent a somewhat restless night. For me, I was really quite calm. I didn't know what to think. I prayed a lot.

On May 5, my doctor showed me the results. I saw what appeared to be a rather large growth in my skull. I felt like I was back in an old nightmare, only this time I might not wake up. From the size of this thing, and the speed of its growth from nothing the year before, it looked ominous. Dr. Lipow, a neurosurgeon, said it could be anything from virulent cancer to scar tissue, to an infection from some unknown source. The latter seemed a likely diagnosis since I had had a left ear infection in March and my ear had begun draining again several weeks prior to the MRI.

I felt a combination of fear, unbelief, and anger. I felt betrayed, by what or whom I didn't identify. I wanted time to finish my book. My sense of being ambushed by fate was very strong.

Strangely enough, I really didn't believe what was happening. I mean, the evidence was before me, I was taking it seriously, but in many ways, it wasn't real. I vowed to go through this with faith, not fear. I had the strength and the will to live, but I was very clear that I didn't want to go on another brain tumor/surgery trip. When thinking of the worst case possibilities—brain surgery, brain cancer, chemotherapy, I didn't want to live.

The next step was an arteriogram to see if there was an extra-large blood supply to this thing. That meant a hospital stay and the repeat of an unpleasant procedure which I remembered quite well. The idea of going through a search and heal process again triggered some fear, but even more anger.

On Monday, May 7, I had an arteriogram. On Tuesday, May 8, Dr. Lipow said there was no extra blood supply to my *thing*, so it wasn't very likely that it was a solid or malignant tumor. He suspected an abscess and said I'd need surgery that week to remove it.

I wanted to wait till I finished revising this book. But he didn't think that was wise or safe. But before setting a definite date for surgery, he was waiting for the report from the hospital's infectious disease department to see if the blood work etc. showed any signs of acute infection throughout my body.

I decided to play it positively (like Annie) and took a walk, praising God and thanking Him for healing me. I put no conditions on the healing, I just acted and thought positively. Within the hour word came that I had no sign of infection anywhere else in my body. If the thing was an infection, it was localized and not threatening my life. At that point, the doctor advised first trying a conservative treatment: antibiotics. Then I would be X rayed again to see if the thing was gone. I was thrilled that I would have the time to complete my research and revision of this book.

I am amazed at how calm I was over the next few weeks. I immersed myself in reading books and articles related to immune function and became more convinced than ever that the mind can cure the body. The fruits of that work are scattered throughout the book. I prayed for a perfect healing.

I discovered a primary seedthought. I was "stewing" over my husband's business problems and heard myself say, "when the (business) crisis came to a head, my new growth was discovered." When I sat down one day to write a history of my husband's business problems, the connection between the two seemed stronger than ever. As I wrote, my ear kept oozing, at a faster rate than at any other time that month. It seems like my emotions connected to my husband's troubles were "stewing around in my head."

On June 3, I went for a CAT scan, filled with hope that all signs of the thing, as I called it, would be gone. The ear drainage had stopped the week before. But immediately after the CAT scan, the drainage began again, and I felt pretty hopeless.

On June 5, I got the result. There was no change from the previous month. The only way to know for sure what was wrong was to go in and look. I thought: "I should be able to heal myself." The alternative—another operation, a biopsy—was horrifying to me.

Lately I've heard criticism of the holistic health movement because people read books like Louise Hay's or Bernie Siegel's, try the techniques, and they don't seem to work. The patient is still sick or even sicker and may feel angry and ripped off. Now, I was facing these same feelings and I had written the book.

I understand first-hand how people feel when they find they haven't cured themselves of some physical problem. I felt like a failure! Despite my beliefs that the process is as important as the end result (in terms of growth and learning), I still felt enormous guilt. "Why couldn't I, of all people (with all my knowledge and self-help practice) cure myself without drugs or surgery?"

What I realized, rather quickly, was that a perfect healing didn't necessarily mean I would be able to avoid surgery. A perfect healing, for me, might mean knowing for sure what caused the thing on the X ray. A perfect healing for me might be to face my fears, have the surgery, and come through easily. I recognized immediately that my biggest fear was "being ambushed," "being caught by surprise," "being unprepared." One part of me expected the best, but a deeper part feared the worst. There it was, the source of, or reason for, my need to worry about everything and to rehearse all kinds of negative scenarios. Now I had a chance to heal that tendency.

I had a core belief that imagining the worst would protect me from the worst. But actually, given what I know about the power of imagination, pretending the worst seems more like praying for the wrong thing than being prepared for it. I realized that I often went to the doctor in hopes of being reassured that I was okay, not really to find a cure for what ailed me. Then, when the doctor did find something wrong (even if it was curable), I often felt ambushed.

I still don't have this whole thing digested and assimilated, but understanding grows within me. Being prepared if the worst happens and still expecting the best is possible. It seems to be related to faith and my recognizing that no matter what, I am a survivor. And whatever will be, will be.

For a month I kept working on this book, completing the revision on July 2, 1989. All the while I used some natural therapies and prayers to heal myself and prepare myself for the inevitable operation. I hoped that the biopsy would show I had a cyst which could be drained easily and I would be done with it. I released my guilt and felt quite certain that what I was going through was the epilog to this book. Somehow, this experience would tie it all together.

On July 5, 1989, I had surgery which was much easier than I expected. I was home the next day. There is no tumor! The surprise diagnosis was a chronic mastoid infection. The mastoid bone looked like a beehive. Just about every cell in the mastoid was filled with infection. Dr. Gill, the ear surgeon, was surprised at how extensive it was, considering that I had had only one ear infection in the previous six months.

While I was enormously relieved that the tumor had not recurred, at first I felt dismay at the thought of months of antibiotic treatment. Evidence of how I dealt with this was my comment to friends, "Antibiotics (a chemical therapy for infection) sure beats chemotherapy for cancer." After several days I made peace with the therapy and became genuinely grateful for how lucky I was.

It is now a year since I began treatment. I've had several rounds of a variety of antibiotics. My ear drainage ceased after several months, with little discomfort. A 1990 MRI brain scan showed improvement from the previous year. And I am more adept at harmonizing my emotions and releasing those worries about which I can do nothing. The problems related to my husband's business are being resolved, and I am part of the solution. I am working hard, feeling happier and healthier than I have in years.

I continue to joyfully receive my perfect healing. Getting rid of an illness, while desirable, is only a part of the healing process. Loving and accepting oneself is as important. Getting rid of fear and releasing the past completes the process. Being able to enjoy life, no matter what, is key. Learning from everything that happens is healthy behavior.

Now, with joy, I share this book with you. Having written it, I understand more about myself, others, psychology, and health. I also have more faith in my ability and God's willingness to provide for me.

I know, though I often forget, that I AM both the observer and the observed, the thoughts and the actions, the words and the deeds, the Creator and the Created. I AM the process of my life. This knowing led to my healing, my mission in life and this book, my testament to the world.

END NOTES
Chapter One

1. Joan Borysenko, *Minding The Body, Mending The Mind,* New York: Bantam Books, 1988, p. 13.
2. ibid. p. 14.
3. ibid. p. 16.
4. Norman Cousins in an excerpt from JAMA, Sept. 16, 1988, Vol. 260 # 11 reprinted in *Noetic Sciences Review,* Winter 1988.
5. Howard and Martha Lewis, *Psychosomatics: How Your Emotions Can Damage Your Health,* New York: Viking Press, 1972, p. 10.
6. Ronald Glasser, M.D., *The Body Is The Hero,* New York: Random House, 1976, p. 228-9.
7. Carolyn Reuben, "AIDS: The Promise of Alternative Treatments" in *East-West Journal,* Sept. 1986, p. 52-66.
8. Buryl Payne, "A Theory of Mind: How We Create Our Reality." (unpublished article).
9. Norman Cousins, *The Healing Heart,* New York: Norton & Co. 1893, p. 200-201.
10. ibid. p. 202.
11. James J. Lynch, *The Broken Heart: The Medical Consequences of Loneliness,* New York: Basic Books 1977, cover flap.
12. Paul Pearsall, Ph.D., *Superimmunity: Master Your Emotions and Improve Your Health,* New York: McGraw-Hill, 1987, p. 112.

Chapter Two
13. James W. Lance, *Headache: Understanding Alleviation,* New York: Scribners, 1975, p. 92.
14. Paul Pearsall, *Superimmunity,* p. 319.
15. *Brain/Mind Bulletin,* Mind/ Hypertension Link, July 1989 p. 2. A review of an article in the *Journal of Nervous and Mental Disease* 177:15-24 by John Sommers-Flanagan and Roger Greenberg.
16. *The Living Bible*—James 3:3-7.

Chapter Three
17. Viktor E. Frankl, M.D., Ph.D., *Man's Search For Meaning: An Introduction to Logotherapy,* Boston: Beacon Press, 1962, p. 65-6.
18. W. C. Ellerbroek, M.D., "Language, Thought and Disease" in *Co-Evolution Quarterly,* Spring 1978, no. 17, p. 38.
19. *Brain/Mind Bulletin,* Vol. 14 # 6, March 1989. Two articles "Experts, Survivors Offer Hope At AIDS Meeting" and "Survivors Beating Odds With Belief, Humor and Self-reliance."
20. Ronald J. Glasser, M.D., *The Body Is The Hero,* back cover.
21. Dennis T. Jaffee, *Healing From Within,* New York: Alfred Knopf p. 122-3, reporting on a study by W. J. Grace and D. T. Graham, "Relationship of Specific Attitudes and Emotions to Certain Bodily Diseases," *Psychosomatic Medicine* 14 (1952): p. 243-51.
22. Milton Ward, *The Brilliant Function Of Pain,* Lakemont, Georgia: CSA Press, 1977, p. 13.
23. The idea for this exercise came from Dennis Jaffeee's *Healing From Within,* p. 124.

Chapter Four
24. Viktor E. Frankl, *Man's Search For Meaning: An Introduction to Logotherapy,* p. 124.

Chapter Five
25.	Tony Schwartz "Doctor Love" in *New York Magazine*, June 12, 1989 p. 42.
26.	James J. Lynch, *The Broken Heart*, p. 57.
27.	Janice K. Kiecolt-Glaser and Ronald Glaser, "Psycological Influences on Immunity: Implications for AIDS," *American Psychologist*, 1988; 43 (11) 892–898.
28.	Paul Pearsall, *Superimmunity*, p. 7.
29.	ibid. p. 9-10.
30.	Barbara B. Brown, Ph.D., *Super Mind: The Ultimate Energy*, New York: Harper & Row, 1980, p. 30-31.

Chapter Six
31.	*Brain/Mind Bulletin*, April 1989, p. 3.
32.	Bernie Siegel, M.D., *Love, Medicine & Miracles*, New York: Harper & Row, 1986, p. 32.

Chapter Eight
33.	Daniel Goleman, Ph.D. *Vital Lies, Simple Truths: The Psychology of Self-Deception*, New York: Simon and Schuster, 1985, p. 90.
34.	Paul Pearsall, *Superimmunity*, p. 19.
35.	ibid. p. 19-20.
36.	George F. Solomon M.D., "The Emerging Field of Psychoneuroimmunology" in *Advances: The Journal For Mind-Body Health*, Institute for the Advancement of Health, Vol. 2 #1, p. 8.

Chapter Nine
37.	Norman Cousins, *The Healing Heart*, p. 204.
38.	Bernie S. Siegel, *Love, Medicine & Miracles*, p. 47.
39.	Daniel Goleman, *Vital Lies, Simple Truths*, p. 89-90.
40.	Ronald J. Glasser, *The Body Is The Hero*, p. 230-237.
41.	Paul Pearsall, *Superimmunity*, p. 10.
42.	David Van Biema, "Learning to Live with a Past That Failed" in *People* magazine, May 29, 1989 p. 79-92. Cover article note, p.4.
43.	Dr. Bernard Lown, introduction to Cousins, *The Healing Heart*, p. 13-16.
44.	John Bradshaw, TV Program #1 in the series The Eight Stages Of Man, "Cradle Hypnosis."

Chapter Ten
45.	Stephen S. Hall, "A Molecular Code Links Emotions, Mind And Health" in *Smithsonian* magazine, June 1989, p. 62-71.
46.	ibid. p. 64.
47.	*The Kripalu Experience Program Guide*, April-Sept. 1988, p. 21.
48.	Tristine Rainer, *The New Diary*, Los Angeles: J. P. Tarcher, 1978, p. 138.

Chapter Eleven
49.	*Brain/Mind Bulletin*, Vol. IV #5, 1979.
50.	*Brain/Mind Bulletin*, Vol. III #7, 1977.
51.	*Brain/Mind Bulletin*, Vol. I #21, 1977, quoting Larry Siegel and William Fleeson of the Institute for Social Rehabilitation and Alan Abrams of Far West Laboratories in San Francisco.
52.	*Brain/Mind Bulletin*, Vol. III #18, 1977-8, a study conducted by dream researcher Henry Reed from *Journal of Clinical Psychology*, 34 (1), p. 150-158.
53.	*Brain/Mind Bulletin*, Vol. V #4, 1980.
54.	*Brain/Mind Bulletin*, Vol. II #14, summarized from an article in *New England Journal of Medicine*, 294, 2, p. 80-84.
55.	*Brain/Mind Bulletin*, Vol. II #7.

56. Justin Stone, *Meditation For Healing!,* New Mexico: Sun Books, 1977, p. 86-87.

Chapter Twelve

57. *Brain/Mind Bulletin,* Vol. IV, Themepack #4, 1979.
58. *Brain/Mind Bulletin,* Vol. XI, Themepack #5, 1987.
59. *Brain/Mind Bulletin,* Vol. XI, Themepack #5, 1987.
60. *Brain/Mind Bulletin,* Vol. VII, Themepack #7, 1982.

Chapter Thirteen

61. *Brain/Mind Bulletin,* Vol. VI, Themepack #7, 1981.
62. *Brain/Mind Bulletin,* Vol. I & II, 1977.
63. Dr. Stephen Aizenstat, interviewed in *Privileged Information* newsletter, Vol. 5, #6, Mar. 1989; "How to Use Dreams."
64. This material was first published in *Dream Network Bulletin.*

Chapter Fourteen

65. *Brain/Mind Bulletin,* Vol. XIII, #8, May 1988, p.2.

APPENDIX: RESOURCES
The following is sampling of the resources available to help you including the addresses and/or phone numbers of some of the health professionals who contributed to this book. They may be right for you. Trust your instincts.

Barbara H. Levine
204 Ridgeview Ave.
Fairfield, CT 06430
203 374-6224

Harry Brown M.D., Psychiatrist
23 White Birch Rd.
Weston, CT 06883
203 226-6670
Workshops and private practice

R. Wallace C. Ellerbroek M.D.,
    (deceased)
    Anyone interested in a more technical, in-depth understanding of Dr. Ellerbroek's treatment program, can read *Language Thought and Disease* in *Perspectives in Biology and Medicine,* Vol. 16, No. 2, Winter 1973. A simpler version appears as *Language, Thought and Disease* in *Co-Evolution Quarterly,* No. 17, Spring 1978.

Erik Esselstyn Ed.D. & Micki Esselstyn
    M.S.W.
Art Of Living Workshops
220 Canner Street
New Haven, CT 06511-2233
203 777-7878

Carl Gruning O.D., Behavioral
    Optometrist
33 Miller Street
Fairfield, CT 06430
203 255-4005
Vision Training.

Alice Katz, Cognitive Therapist
13 High Point Rd.
Westport CT 06880
203 259 8026
Compulsive eating and anger issues.

Bob Lang M.D., Endocrinologist,
    Internist
4699 Main Street
Bridgeport CT 06606.
203 372-7715
Specialist in *Healing Conversations.*

Robert Marshall D.C., Chiropractor
40 Red Coat Rd.
Westport CT 06880
203 226-6366

Emmett Miller M.D.
c/o Source Cassette Learning Systems,
    Inc.
P. O. Box W
Stanford, CA 94305
415 328-7171

Buryl Payne
c/o Psycho-Physics Labs
P.O. Box 697
Hanalei, Hawaii, 96714
Tapes on dreamwork and world peace;
    magnetic healing

Jacqueline Ruzga D.C., Chiropractor
2452 Black Rock Turnpike
Fairfield, CT 06430
203 372-7333

Marvin Schweitzer N.D., Naturopath
c/o Center For Holistic Medicine
71 East Ave.
Norwalk, CT 06851
203 838-9355

Bernie Siegel M.D.
c/o ECAP (Exceptional Cancer Patients,
    Inc.)
1302 Chapel St.
New Haven, CT 06511
203 865-8392
    ECAP groups help patients with all serious-chronic illnesses. ECAP trains health professionals. For an information packet including referrals to regional ECAP-like support groups and a schedule of Bernie's lectures and workshops, send $5 dollars. Free catalogue of tapes, videos and books.

Roberta Tager
104 Imperial Ave.
Westport, CT 06880
203 222-7507
Synergistic Therapy: integrates Rohun,
    Reiki & MariEl.

Dorothy Thau, Health Counselor
19 Saugatuck River Road
Weston, CT 06883
203 226-1908
Holistic healing, private consultations.

Montague Ullman M.D., Psychiatrist
55 Orlando Ave.
Ardsley, N Y 10502
For information about dream workshops.

Linda Zelizer, Hypnotherapist
c/o Center For Personal Development
514 Giordano Drive
Yorktown Heights, NY 10598
914 962-4397
Workshops, private practice, consultant
to business on human relations skills.

Inclusion on the following list of people or groups doing work in related fields doesn't mean a blanket endorsement, but that I have found something of value in their work.

Deborah Lueth Aikens
185 Alexander Ave.
Redwood City, CA 94061
415 367-9817
Stress management consultant to
business.

American Chiropractic Association
2200 Grand Ave.
Des Moines, IA 50312
800 368-3083

Association for Research and
Enlightenment (ARE)
P.O. Box 595
Virginia Beach, VA 23451
800 368-2727
Edgar Cayce Foundation —Membership
info and catalogue.

Brain/Mind Bulletin
Marilyn Ferguson, Publisher
Box 42211
Los Angeles, CA 90042, USA
(U.S. $35/year, 12 issues.) For
complimentary issue send self-
addressed business-sized envelope.

Buddhism of Nichiren Daishonin
c/o N.S.A. World Tribune
525 Wilshire Blvd.
Santa Monica, CA 90406, USA
213 451-8811
Weekly newspaper: information about
American Buddhism.

Roslyn Bruyere
Healing Light Center Church
204 East Wilson
Glendale, CA 91206
Newsletter *The Light Bearer;* Healing,
Classes.

The Giraffe Project
John Graham, Executive Director
Box 759
Langley Wa. 98260
206 221-7989
"People who stick their necks out for the
common good."

Gerson Institute
P. O. Box 430
Bonita, California 92002
619 267-1150
Detoxifying to heal cancer and other
chronic illnesses.

Louise Hay
c/o Hay House
P.o. Box 2212
Santa Monica, CA 90406
213 394-7445
Lectures, Books, Tapes, Groups.

Institute for The Advancement of Health
16 East 53rd St.
New York, NY 10022
212 832-8282
*Advances: The Journal for mind-body
health..* Latest scientific knowledge
reported on to further the study of
mind-body interactions and their use in
healing.

Institute For Noetic Sciences
475 Gate Five Road
Suite 300
Sausalito, CA 94965
415 331-3650
Research & education in human
consciousness; Journal.

Kripalu Center For Yoga And Health
Box 793
Lenox, MA 01240
413 637 3280
Retreat, classes, medical evaluations,
    private sessions

Acharya Sushil Kumar, Muni Ji
c/o Siddhachalam
R.D. #4 Box 374
Blairstown, NJ 07825
201 362-9793
Classes in Jain philosphy, non-violence,
    healing, chanting

College of Optometrists in Vision
    Development
P.O. Box 285
Chula Vista, CA 92012
For names of Functional-Behavioral
    Optometrists.

Paul Solomon
Fellowship of The Inner Light
620 14th St.
Virginia Beach, VA 23451
Newsletter *Supportive Lifestyles.*
    Catalogue, classes.

Siddha Yoga Dham (SYDA)
P. O. Box 600
South Fallsburg, NY 12779
914 434-2000
Retreats, courses, books, tapes and
    meditation supplies.

S.T.A.R. Foundation (Space, Technology
    & Research)
Richard Smolowe & Greta Woodrew
448 Rabbit Skin Road
Waynesville, NC 28786
Newsletter *The Woodrew Update*
    Healing and survival

Jo Willard
President of Natural Hygiene Inc.
P.O. Box 2132
Huntington, CT 06484
203 929-1557
Journal - Sample copy and Catalogue
    Research Dept. for any health related
    subject. Personal consultations.

TRAININGS FOR PERSONAL GROWTH AND TRANSFORMATION

Werner Erhard & Associates
765 California Street
San Francisco, Calif. 94108
415 951-2222
The *est* training has been replaced by a
    new basic program called The Forum.

Human Potential Network Inc.
Womanspirit Course
Suite 2J
115 Fourth Ave.
New York, NY 10003
212 353-0808
Inner healing therapist Harriet Salinger.

Insight Transformational Seminars
2101 Wilshire Blvd.
Santa Monica, CA 90403
213 829-9816
Seminars, books, tapes. Insights is an
    arm of:
The Movement of Spiritual Inner
    Awareness
MSIA — PO Box 3935
Los Angeles, CA 90051
Spiritual Courses and *The Movement
    Newspaper*

PRAYER LINE PHONE NUMBERS AND ADDRESSES

Call and a prayer counselor will pray with you at no cost, though you are welcome to contribute. Christian groups will pray with you regardless of your religion. I do not necessarily agree with all the beliefs of these groups, but have found them personally helpful at many different times. I called or wrote them for prayer, prior to my brain surgery.

Abundant Life Prayer Group
Oral and Richard Roberts
Tulsa, OK 74171
918 495-7777
24 hour prayer line; City of Faith Medical and Research Center; Oral Roberts University. Literature and Tapes.

Kenneth Copeland Ministries
Fort Worth, TX 76192
Written prayer requests; magazine *Voice of Victory.*

Church Of White Eagle Lodge
P.O. Box 8182
The Woodlands, TX 77387
Absentee healing, books and tapes, retreats, and workshops.

Grace N' Vessels of Christ Ministry
77 Grays Bridge Road
Brookfield, CT 06804
203 775-1990
24 hour prayer line, newsletter, musical healing services.

Jewish Voice Broadcasts
PO Box 6
Phoenix, AR 85001
602 867-8700
Prophetic Magazine; TV and Radio Shows, Prayer Hotline.

Jimmy Swaggart Ministries
PO Box 2550
Baton Rouge, LA 70821
504 768-7000
Prayer Line 5AM to 5PM, books, tapes, magazine.

Kolel America
132 Nassau Street
New York, NY 10038
1-800-545-PRAY.
Jewish Hotline for Prayer for your request at the Wailing Wall in Israel. Kolel America is the American Charity of Rabbi Meir Baal Haness.

Mike Evans Ministries
PO Box 709
Bedford, TX 76021
Write for prayer; catalog of books and tapes.

New Covenant Church
Box 690788
Orlando, FL 32869
Inspiration from people who carry on no matter what.

Robert Schuller, Hour of Power
Garden Grove, CA
714 NEW-HOPE (639-4673)
24 hour prayer line, counseling and literature.

700 Club—Pat Robertson
Virginia Beach, VA 23463
804 420-0700
24 hour prayer line, counseling, books & tapes.

Silent Unity
Unity Village, MO 64065
816 246-5400
24 hour prayer line, books, tapes, monthly prayer magazine *The Daily Word.*

Rev. Willard Fuller
Lively Stones Healing Fellowship
P. O. Box 2007
Palatka, FL 32077
904 649-9288
Healing services; classes and retreats; books and tapes.

Zola Levitt Ministries
Jewish Believers in Christ
PO Box 12268
Dallas, TX 75225
Newsletter, Tapes, TV Program, Tours to Israel.

RECOMMENDED READING

Advances: The Journal for Mind/Body Health. New York: Institute for Advancement of Health.

American International Reiki Association. *The Reiki Journal.* 2210 Wilshire Blvd., Suite 831, Santa Monica, CA 90403.

Atkins, Dr. Robert. *Dr. Atkins Health Revolution: How Complementary Medicine can Extent Your Life* New York: Houghton-Mifflin, 1988

Bird, Chistopher and Tompkins, Peter. *The Secret Life of Plants.* New York: Harper and Row, 1973.

Blythe, Peter. *Self-Hypnotism: Its Power and Practice.* Ontario, Canada: Coles Publishing Co., 1978.

Bondi, Julia A. *Lovelight: Unveiling the Mysteries of Sex and Romance.* New York: Pocket Books, 1989.

Borysenko, Joan Ph.D. *Minding the Body, Mending the Mind.* New York: Bantam, 1988.

Brown, Barbara B. Ph.D. *Super Mind: The Ultimate Energy.* New York: Harper & Row, 1980

Bruce, Shelly. *Tomorrow is Today.* Indianapolis: Bobbs-Merrill, 1983.

Church, Dawson. *Communing With the Spirit of Your Unborn Child.* Boulder Creek, CA: Aslan Pub., 1988.

Church, Dawson and Sherr, Dr. Alan. *The Heart of the Healer.* Boulder Creek, CA: Aslan Pub., 1988.

Cousins, Norman. *Anatomy of an Illness as Percieved by the Patient.* New York: W.W. Norton, 1979.

Cousins, Norman. *The Healing Heart: Antidotes to Panic and Helplessness* New York: W.W. Norton, 1983.

Desowitz, Robert S. Ph.D. *The Thorn in the Starfish: The Immune System & How it Works.* New York: W. W. Norton, 1987.

Dream Network Bulletin. 670 East Rio Rd., Charlottesville VA 22901.

Egan, Gerard. "Logos: Man's Translation of Himself into Language" in Joseph DeVito, *Language: Concept and Processes.* Englewood Cliffs, NJ: Prentice-Hall, 1973.

Evans, Mike. *The Return.* New York: Thomas Nelson, 1986.

Ferguson, Marilyn. *Brain/Mind Bulletin.* Monthly, Box 42211, Los Angeles CA 90042.

Foundation For Inner Peace. *A Course in Miracles.* c/o PO Box 635 Tiburon, CA 94920,1975.

Frankl, Viktor B. *Man's Search For Meaning: An Introduction To Logotherapy.* Boston: Beacon Press, 1962.

Freeman, Joel. *God Is Not Fair: Coming to Terms with Life's Raw Deals.* PO Box 1576, San Bernadino, CA 92402, 1987.

Fuller, Elizabeth. *The Touch of Grace.* New York: Dodd, Mead, 1986.

Friedlander, Mark and Phillips, Terry. *Winning the War Within.* Emmaus, PA: Rodale Press, 1986.

Gawain, Shakti. *Creative Visualization.* New World Library., Mill Valley, CA, 1978.

Gerson, Max, M.D. *A Cancer Therapy.* PO Box 1035 Del Mar, CA 92014: Totality Books, 1975.

Glasser, Ronald J., M.D. *The Body Is the Hero.* New York: Random House, 1976.

Glasser, William. *Positive Addiction.* New York: Harper & Row, 1976.

Goleman, Daniel. *The Varieties of the Meditative Experience.* New York: Irvington, 1977.

Goleman, Daniel. *Vital Lies, Simple Truths: The Psychology of Self-Deception.* New York: Simon and Schuster, 1985.

Halacy, D.S. *Man and Memory: Breakthroughs in the Science of the Human Mind.* New York: Harper & Row, 1970.

Halpern, Steven, Ph.D. *Tuning the Human Instrument*. 1775 Old Country Road, #19, Belmont, CA 94002: Spectrum Research Institute, 1978.

Hay, Louise L. *You Can Heal Your Life*. Hay House Inc. P.O. Box 2212, Santa Monica, CA 90406, 1987.

Hunt, Morton. *The Universe Within: A New Science Explores the Human Mind*. New York: Simon and Schuster, 1982.

Institute of Noetic Sciences. *Noetic Sciences Review*. 475 Gate Five Road, Suite 300, Sausalito, CA 94965.

Jaffee, Dennis T., Ph.D. *Healing From Within*. New York: Alfred Knopf, 1980.

King, Lester S. *The Growth of Medical Thought*. Chicago: University of Chicago Press, 1963.

Koestler, Arthur. *The Lotus and the Robot*. New York: Macmillan, 1961.

Koestler, Arthur. *The Ghost in the Machine*. New York: Macmillan, 1967.

Lance, James W. *Headache: Understanding Alleviation*. New York: Schribners, 1975.

LeCron, Leslie M. *Self-Hypnotism*. New York: New American Library, 1964.

Lewis, Howard R. and Martha E. *Psychosomatics: How Your Emotions Can Damage Your Health*. New York: Viking, 1972.

Lynch, James J. *The Broken Heart: The Medical Consequences of Loneliness*. New York: Basic Books, 1977.

Miller, Emmett, M.D., and Lueth, Deborah, Ph.D. *Self Imagery*. Berkeley: Celestial Arts, 1986.

Pearsall, Paul, Ph.D. *Superimmunity: Master Your Emotions & Improve Your Health*. New York: McGraw-Hill, 1987.

Pelletier, Kenneth. *Mind as Healer, Mind as Slayer*. New York: Dell, 1977.

Postman, Neil. *Crazy Talk, Stupid Talk*. New York: Delacorte Press, 1976.

Rainer, Tristine. *The New Diary*. Los Angeles: J.P. Tarcher, 1978.

Reed, Henry. *Dream Realizations: A Dream Incubation Workbook*. 503 Lake Drive, Virginia Beach, VA 23451, 1984.

Reuben, Carolyn. "Aids: The Promise of Alternative Treatments," pp. 52–66. *East West Journal*. Sept., 1986.

Roger, John and McWilliams, Peter. *You Can't Afford the Luxury of a Negative Thought*. Box 69773, Los Angeles, CA 90069: Prelude Press, 1988.

Rosanoff, Nancy. *Intuition Workout: A Practical Guide to Discovering and Developing Your Inner Knowing*. Boulder Creek, CA: Aslan Publishing, 1988.

Rosenbaum, Jean M.D. *The Mind Factor: How Your Emotions Affect Your Health*. Englewood Cliffs, NJ: Prentice-Hall, 1973.

Siegel, Bernie S. M.D. *Love, Medicine & Miracles*. New York: Harper & Row, 1986.

Siegel, Bernie S. M.D. *Peace, Love & Healing*. New York: Harper & Row, 1989.

Silva, Jose. *The Silva Mind Control Method*. Pocket Books, 1977.

Simonton, Carl. *Getting Well Again: A Step by Step Self-Help Guide to Overcoming Cancer for Patients and Their Families*. Los Angeles: J.P. Tarcher, 1978.

Smithsonian Magazine. 900 Jefferson Drive, Washington, DC 20560.

Sontag, Susan. *Illness as Metaphor*. New York: Farrar, Straus & Giroux, 1977.

Steincrohn, Peter J. M.D. and LaFia, David, M.D. *How to Master Your Nerves*. New York: Cowles, 1970.

Stone, Christopher. *Re-Creating Your Self*. P.O. Box 10616, Portland, OR 97210: Metamorphous Press.

Stone, Justin F. *Meditation For Healing!* P.O. Box 4383, Albuquerque, NM 87106: Sun Publishing, 1977.

The Woodrew Update. S.T.A.R. Foundation, 448 Rabbit Skin Road, Waynesville, NC 28786.

Ullman, Montague, M.D. and Zimmerman, Nan. *Working With Dreams.* Los Angeles: J.P. Tarcher, 1979.

Ullman, Montague, M.D. and Linner, Claire. *The Variety of Dream Experience.* New York: Continuum Publishers, 1987.

Vlahos, Olivia. *Body: The Ultimate Symbol.* New York: Lippincott, 1979.

Wallace, Amy and Henkin, Bill. *The Psychic Healing Book.* New York: Dell, 1978.

Ward, Milton. *The Brilliant Function of Pain.* NY: Optimus Books, c/o CSA Press, Lakemont, GA, 1977.

Westlake, Aubrey T. *The Pattern of Health.* Berkeley: Shambhala, 1973.

White Eagle. Books on healing, spiritual growth. Liss, Hampshire, England: White Eagle Publishing Trust.

Personal Power Cards   by Barbara Gress

Personal Power Cards is a simple, easy to use set of
flash cards for emotional wellness. Each set includes
55 cards, a carrying pouch, and an 80 page booklet.
The Cards help retrain your feelings to be positive
and healthy. Their combination of colors, shapes,
and words allows positive thoughts to penetrate deep
into your subconscious, "programming" your emotions for health.

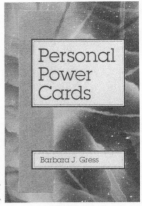

"In the twenty years I have been using color and mind
imagery with patients, I have never seen any approach
have such a great benefit on self-discipline and self-
esteem. "

—Richard Shames, M.D., Family Practitioner
and author of *Healing with Mind Power*

$18.95

Intuition Workout   by Nancy Rosanoff

This practical training manual teaches simple techniques to access our deepest sources of inner knowing
in any situation.

    The author, one of America's outstanding corpo-
rate trainers, shows that intuition, like a muscle, is
strengthened by training. She outlines dozens of case
histories and step-by-step exercises proven effective
even with "non-intuitive" people.

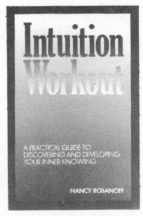

    "A workout in cultivating our inner resources and
building self-confidence. Once you know how to do
it, you can adapt the techniques to any situation."
—*New York Daily News*

Available as a book or audio tape.
Also sold as a set for a $3 discount.

$9.95 book or tape

Soul Return   by Aminah Raheem

Expertly blending Western psychology with eastern traditions, Soul Return presents a scientific and well-
reasoned survey of the role factors like love, wisdom,
service, and enlightenment play in optimal health. Dr.
Raheem gently guides us into finding our deeper purposes before trying to fix physical or mental ailments.

    An ultra-clear explanation of the role that spirituality
should play in psychology, Soul Return presents a com-
pelling case for returning the soul to a place of primary
causation when dealing with our bodies, minds, and
emotions.

    Blending both good psychology and deep spirituality,
this profoundly important book re-introduces mind to
spirit.

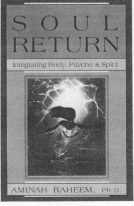

$12.95

The Heart of the Healer
Edited by Dawson Church & Dr. Alan Sherr

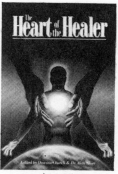

A collection of outstanding figures on the leading edge of conventional and holistic medicine, including Bernie Siegel, Norman Cousins and Prince Charles, draw on their deepest personal experiences to explore how we get in touch with the essence of wellness. This classic has been called "Exceptional" —*SSC Booknews*; "Thought-provoking" —*Publisher's Weekly*; "Profound...provocative" —*Ram Dass*.

$14.95

Voice Power
by Dr. Joan Kenley

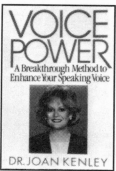

The sound of your voice can have more than five times the impact of the words you say. *Voice Power* shows you how to draw on the resources of your whole body to release your natural voice—the voice that is truly and fully you. It shows you how to integrate the deepest roots of your personality, your vitality and your sexuality, to project charisma and confidence.

"...a fun read as well as a very practical, thorough book." —*Network Magazine*

$18.95 Hardback

Love is a Secret
by Andrew Vidich

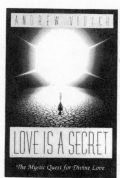

What is God's love and how do we experience it. Drawing on the words of saints and scholars from a rich variety of religious traditions, from Taoism to Christianity, from Sufism to Judaism, this book illuminates the psychology of humankind's deepest spiritual experiences.

"In a world yearning to find its unity and connectedness, this book invokes for all to hear, 'Love has only a beginning, my friend; it has no ending.' " —*Dr Arthur Stein, Professor Peace Studies, Univ. of R.I.*

$9.95

The Unmanifest Self
by Ligia Dantes

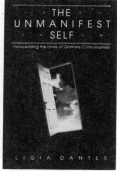

This book, like a warm, gentle friend, guides us toward an experience of self-transformation that is quite different from our usual waking consciousness, that is vastly more than an improved version of the old self. *The Unmanifest Self* teaches us the art of *objective self-observation*, a powerful tool to separate the essential truth of who we are from the labyrinth of thoughts and emotions in which we are often caught.

"...beautiful and inspiring." —*Willis Harmon*

$9.95

Order Form

(Please print legibly)   Date ——————————

Name ——————————————————————————

Address ————————————————————————

City ———————————— State ——— Zip ——————

Phone ——————————————————————————

Please send a catalog to my friend:

Name ——————————————————————————

Address ————————————————————————

City ———————————— State ——— Zip ——————

Quantity Discounts!

$2 off if you order 2 items
$3 off if you order 3 items
$4 off if you order 4 items, etc...

Item	Qty.	Price	Amount
Personal Power Cards		$18.95	
Intuition Workout (book)		$9.95	
Intuition Workout (tape)		$9.95	
Soul Return		$12.95	
The Heart of the Healer		$14.95	
Voice Power (hardback book)		$18.95	
Love is a Secret		$9.95	
The Unmanifest Self		$9.95	
		Subtotal	
		Quantity Discount	
		Calif. res. add 6.5% sales tax	
		Shipping	
		Grand Total	

Add for shipping:
Book Rate: $2.00 for first item, $1.00 for ea. add. item
First Class/UPS: $4.00 for first item, $2.00 ea. add. item
Foreign: Double shipping rates

Check type of payment:

☐ Check or money order enclosed

☐ VISA   ☐ MasterCard

Acct. # ——————————————————

Exp. Date ——————————————

Signature ——————————————

Send order to:
**Aslan Publishing
310 Blue Ridge Drive
Boulder Creek, CA 95006**

or call to order:
**(408) 338-7504
(800) 372-3100**   YBB

Order Form

(Please print legibly)　　　　　Date ————————

Name ——————————————————————————

Address ————————————————————————

City ——————————— State ——— Zip ——————

Phone ————————————————————————————

Please send a catalog to my friend:

Name ——————————————————————————

Address ————————————————————————

City ——————————— State ——— Zip ——————

Quantity Discounts!

$2 off if you order 2 items
$3 off if you order 3 items
$4 off if you order 4 items, etc...

Item	Qty.	Price	Amount
Personal Power Cards		$18.95	
Intuition Workout (book)		$9.95	
Intuition Workout (tape)		$9.95	
Soul Return		$12.95	
The Heart of the Healer		$14.95	
Voice Power (hardback book)		$18.95	
Love is a Secret		$9.95	
The Unmanifest Self		$9.95	
Subtotal			
Quantity Discount			
Calif. res. add 6.5% sales tax			
Shipping			
Grand Total			

Add for shipping:
Book Rate: $2.00 for first item, $1.00 for ea. add. item
First Class/UPS: $4.00 for first item, $2.00 ea. add. item
Foreign: Double shipping rates

Check type of payment:

☐ Check or money order enclosed

☐ VISA　　☐ MasterCard

Acct. # ————————————————

Exp. Date ————————————————

Signature ————————————————

Send order to:
Aslan Publishing
310 Blue Ridge Drive
Boulder Creek, CA 95006

or call to order:
(408) 338-7504
(800) 372-3100　　　YBB